T0096098

PRAISE FOR *THE GOOD SH*T*

"You are the person who is most in touch with your own body. You need to take onus for your own life and be responsible for yourself. Dr. Sinett is helping people everywhere understand the signs of their bodies and the importance of their poop to help increase the prevention and early detection of colorectal cancer, the number two cause of cancer death in both sexes. Life is precious. Read this book and start paying attention to the vital information the toilet is telling you." —**DR. JOHN PROCACCINO**, MD, FACS, FASCRS, Director of Colon and Rectal Services for Central Region, Chief of Colon and Rectal Surgery for North Shore Hospital, Director of Colorectal Fellowship

"As dietitians, we are often focused on what you're putting in your body, but what comes out can be a sign about what you should and shouldn't be eating. Dr. Sinett's book is a needed reminder that your digestive system is like your fingerprint, specific to you, and the newest fad diet may not work with your microbiome. *The Good Sh*t* can help you lose weight *and* feel great by achieving your own optimal gut health." —**DEBORAH MALKOFF-COHEN**, MS, RD, CDN, CDE

"Dr. Sinett takes a holistic approach to understanding how our gastrointestinal issues may be related to the food we eat and the way we feel from head to toe. This book clears up the messages our own bodies are sending and gives us the tools we need to normalize our own digestive systems!" —**DR. ALEXANDRA KREPS**, MD, Tru Whole Care and Mount Sinai

"The form, character, and frequency of one's bowel movements are important clues to intestinal health. When evaluating patients, I routinely question them about their bowel habits in order to determine the most appropriate diagnostic and treatment plan. Dr. Sinett's book allows you at home to analyze your own bowel movements and make important realizations about your own health! *The Good Sh*t* will likely lead many to get a colonoscopy and could prevent colon cancer in many readers!" —**DR. KEN MILLER**, MD, Gastroenterologist, Clinical Instructor, Mount Sinai Hospital

"Finally, a common sense approach to diets! There is nothing more confusing than hearing conflicting 'Eat this, not that!' advice. Biochemically, we are all different, and Dr. Sinett shows how your diet should be unique to you. Dr. Sinett explains it all here in easily digestible terms and makes a potentially 'shitty' topic actually fun and attainable!" —**LANA BUTNER**, N.D., L.Ac

THE Good Sh*t

What Your Sh*t Tells You About What You Should or Shouldn't Eat

DR. TODD SINETT

EAST END PRESS
BRIDGEHAMPTON • NEW YORK

THE GOOD SHIT:

What Your Sh*t Tells You About

What You Should or Shouldn't Eat

Published by

EAST END PRESS

Bridgehampton, NY

ISBN: 978-1-7324912-9-8

Ebook ISBN: 978-1-7345268-0-6

First Edition

Book Design by Neuwirth & Associates

Cover Design by Neuwirth & Associates

Manufactured in the United States of America

10 9 8 7 6 5 4 3 2 1

This book is dedicated to my mom, who has filled my life with good shit. She is calm and sensible, and always balances my father's whims—like the time she convinced him to return his impulse purchase of a Corvette and get a good family car instead. She is cool under pressure—she once successfully performed the Heimlich when my son choked on a piece of steak. She is brave—more than I ever can be as she undergoes her fight with colon cancer—and is my inspiration for this book. Nothing makes me happier than when she says, "Todd, don't be a pain!"

• Contents •

THE Good Sh*t

Introduction

To Be Truly Healthy, You Must Examine Your Shit!

After working with patients for over twenty years, I have reached the conclusion that everything that we thought we knew about nutrition is wrong. I have watched trend after trend, diet after diet, without any true lasting benefits or consensus. The extremes of diets seem to be worsening as people increasingly try to look their best.

But restrictive fad diets have not helped us, as a society, eat any more healthfully or have a healthier relationship with food. They may have helped us shed some weight, but, by and large, haven't helped us keep it off for good.

One of the major problems with fad diets is that new, compelling information that comes out is often refuted years later. In recent years, it seems we have been in The Battle of the Diets: low fat versus high fat, dairy versus dairy-free, gluten versus gluten-free, paleo versus vegan. We've been told to have frequent small meals all throughout the day and then heard we should go days with barely eating, except for juices! We are told only to eat fruits or vegetables and then we hear someone who says we should be avoiding them altogether! All of this information and misinformation has left people downright confused.

As I watched all of these theories come and go over the last decade, I would frequently ask myself, "How can two diametrically opposed diets both declare the same types of success? Shouldn't one be the consensus winner and the other a consensus loser?" It left me confused as to which was right and which was wrong, and which I should be following myself or recommending to patients in my practice who seemed to suffer from diet-related back pain and other issues. They all made compelling arguments, with dieters sharing personal stories of life transformations, including weight loss, more energy, and even more Instagram followers!

I finally realized one important thing: *The only consensus in all diets is that there is no consensus!* For every diet, there is an equal and opposite diet.

You Must Examine Your Shit!

So how do you make sense of any of this conflicting bullshit? How do you know what you should and shouldn't be eating?

The answer to this question would elude me for years until I decided to clean up my diet with a New Year's resolution to go on a real health kick. Even though I don't drink alcohol or coffee or indulge in a lot of sweets, I wanted to improve my diet: no more sweets or simple carbohydrates for me! I cut out my morning bagel and decided I was going to have high-fiber oatmeal every day for breakfast, a salad for lunch, and lean proteins for dinner. After a week on this diet, I was hoping to notice a difference in my energy levels and overall well-being. The changes that I experienced in just one week were mind-blowing to me. Yes, my energy levels changed—as did my sense of well-being. However, both got *significantly worse*. I had a dramatic increase in bloating and stomach pain, alternating bouts of constipation and diarrhea, and by the end of the week, my neck, shoulders, and upper back got so tight I could barely turn my head or bend. I asked myself, "Could it actually be possible that the change in my diet was the cause of my pain and suffering?"

I immediately returned to my old eating habits, which had been pretty healthy to begin with. Within two days, I felt significantly better. What I experienced in just a short time led me to a whole new understanding of nutrition. Could it be that oatmeal or salads were less healthy than a bagel or a sandwich? For me, I would say the answer is yes. I understand that a bagel may be less nutritious than oatmeal; however, my body digested and functioned better when eating a bagel for breakfast than when eating oatmeal. My body reacted well to a turkey sandwich, but after eating salad I would feel gassy and bloated, resulting in diarrhea.

This led me to a new question. *What is healthy for me?* and *What is healthy for you?*

This was my *aha* moment. There isn't one right diet for everyone! Some people function better eating more proteins, while others function better having more carbohydrates. Some feel great going long times between meals, while others need to eat every three hours. Some people can handle dairy, some are lactose intolerant. Some function quite well on breads and grains, while others are gluten sensitive. Eating oatmeal every day for five days adversely affected my health, but a bagel with peanut butter kept me feeling great. *Everyone is unique, and what may be healthy for some could be unhealthy for others.*

So, whether you eat a "healthy" diet or an "unhealthy" diet, whether you are "vegan" or eat "paleo," whether you start your day with a green drink or an eighteen-ounce cup of coffee, whether you eat pizza or salad for lunch, your diet needs to be healthy for *you* and *your digestive system*, and everyone's intestines are a little bit different. This explains why opposite diets can tout the same successes. It is not a case of one diet being right and the other being wrong—they are both right and both wrong. Now all we need to do is figure which diet is uniquely right or healthy for you.

But how do you know if your diet is right or wrong for you? How can you choose a diet relatively quickly without spending years sifting through the fads?

While sitting on the toilet bowl, I had a revelation. The common denominator on how I felt was answered in my shit! When I was feeling good, I was having good healthy bowel movements, and when I wasn't, I was having either diarrhea or hardened pellets. A breakfast of oatmeal left me gassy and constipated, but eggs, cold cereal, or a bagel didn't impact me that way. Spicy foods and large salads would give me diarrhea but not a sandwich or blander foods. A good bowel movement is your body's message of a job well done. Simply put: If you are having good, healthy bowel movements, then your body is ridding yourself of your waste products properly. If your body is ridding you of waste products properly, then what you are putting into your mouth is good for your digestive system. If you are eating foods good for your digestive system, you reap a plethora of benefits, like reduced muscle pain, less bloating, gas, and other stomach complaints, more energy, and less build-up. All of this can translate into fewer pounds! It can also translate into something much bigger, like reduced risk of cancer and premature death!

IT'S THE OUTPUT THAT'S REALLY IMPORTANT!

Could it be that we have been focusing on the wrong end this entire time? We have been studying what we have been eating (i.e., input) this entire time with little to no regard for how our body is processing the foods and excreting them (i.e., the output). I believe that what you are consuming is way less important than what you are digesting and handling, and that we have hyper-focused on food when we should be focused on poop!

I find some people have trouble, er, digesting this information! It is hard to train your mind to think differently than what we've learned from the fads. But think of it like this: Evaluating your health based on your food choices is like studying for an exam and hoping you will get the answers correct on the test. If you prefer to approach the issue using the scientific method, food choices and diet are the hypothesis and your shit is the results, or the conclusion! Evaluating your diet through your shit is essentially having the answer key!

With The Good Shit Diet, I am not encouraging you to throw out common sense but rather to embrace it. Are your food choices important for your health? Of course they are! It is just that food choices have been overly emphasized and scrutinized. To me, the most important aspect in proper digestion and diet is the quality of your shit.

LET YOUR SHIT GUIDE YOU

In this book, you will learn about the digestive system and how your body talks. You'll learn how to wade through all the diet bullshit that hasn't worked for you and never will. You'll learn how to figure out which foods are affecting your output and how to best create a nutrition plan that works for you and for the way your body functions. You will learn what a good shit is, what it should look like, and how to have them regularly, so that you can start looking and feeling better. This book is a path to self-discovery that will open your eyes to specific foods that you digest and excrete well, as well as others that you should be staying away from—even if they have been described as a supposed "superfood." Ultimately, this is a book about how to have really great shits. Let's get down to business!

1

Shit Talk

I'm Not Shitting You! Poop Matters!

For some reason, discussing poop is taboo—even more so than talking about sex and nudity! Very often, people will only poop in their own homes. In a new relationship? The fear of having to poop when you are with your new significant other is terrifying! Poop, however, is just a bodily function. We all do it, and it's as much a part of being healthy as exercise is! It's time we start talking about shit and the way having a good shit, regularly, can improve your health.

Are you still skeptical that your poop could be the answer to your weight problems or pain? Let's compare your diet to high-performance gasoline for race cars. Gasoline developers look to create the right formulation of fuel, which is then put to the test. If the car performs well, the chemists know that their gasoline formula was correct, but if the car breaks down, stalls, or doesn't run optimally, the fuel wasn't correct.

The same concept goes for humans. "People can tell a measure of their health by their bowel movement," says Ted Loftness, MD, an internist in Litchfield, Minnesota. Ashkan Farhadi, MD, a gastroenterologist at Orange Coast Memorial Medical Center and director of MemorialCare Medical Group's Digestive Disease Project in Fountain Valley, California, agrees. "Our bowel movements are the result of so many processes in the body." Basically, if something is out of whack in your body, there's a decent chance your poop is going to tell you about it.

YOUR BODY SPEAKS

How do you know if you are full? Your body tells you.

How do you know if your body is too toxic? Your skin may break out.

How do you know if you are drinking the right amount of water? The color of your pee tells you! (If it looks like apple juice, you need more and if it is clear you are hydrated.)

How do you know if you are eating and digesting well?

Shit Talk

A good, healthy shit will tell you!

LISTEN TO YOUR SHIT

Body language isn't just a tool to interpret someone's emotions: It is a vital piece of information telling you how your own body is functioning. Our Western society has been ignoring our body's language for far too long. Pain, for example, is your body telling you that there is a problem. Pain is your body's protective mechanism, and without your ability to experience pain, you would do some serious harm to your body. Yet when we are in pain, we want to dismiss the pain as quickly as possible without trying to learn why we are in pain in the first place. Very often, taking a pain medication is our immediate response to feeling pain, but that just masks the symptoms for several hours. Taking pain medication in this way is analogous to removing the battery of a smoke alarm because the alarm is too loud—regardless of whether there is a fire or not. There are plenty of stomach medications, both over-the-counter and prescription-based, that will allow you to override your body's messaging so that you can eat some of your favorite foods. In fact, there's an entire generation that will answer the question "How do you spell relief?" with "R-o-l-a-i-d-s!" Marketing has gotten us all to turn to Rolaids instead of dealing with the real issue: our food choices and our corresponding poop! It's why $1.3 billion is spent every year on laxatives, $263 million on anti-diarrheal medicines, and $2.6 billion on heartburn medications (https://www.chpa.org/OTCsCategory.aspx). Those numbers have steadily risen over the last several years. These growing sales are a sign that more and more people are ignoring their poop.

But our excrement is a key way in which our bodies speak. If your body doesn't like dairy, it shouldn't be fed dairy in the first place, lactose pill or not. If you need an antacid to eat a spicy bowl of chili, you should pass on the spice and prepare a milder recipe.

UNDERSTANDING INPUT

To understand the concept of our output being a language all its own, we first need to start at the beginning with food. It's essential to establish a new way of looking at food and realize foods are essentially neutral, consisting of both good and bad.

What does this mean exactly? It's like my bagel versus the oatmeal. For others, it may be choosing chicken wings or broccoli. Chicken wings might not be the "healthier" choice, but for some, broccoli can be an undigestible, stomach-upsetting food; whereas chicken wings could get broken down into energy and waste products that are excreted properly. It isn't healthy if you are eating a kale salad with lemon and chia seeds if it creates a bad poop or causes you to feel gassy and bloated every time you eat it. This ties back to how we get success stories from a variety of opposing diets. Some bodies are not meant to digest gluten. So, low-carb plans are better for those particular people and lead to more energy, better poops that rid the body of bloat, and an overall feeling of better well-being. Some bodies can't tolerate too many raw fruits and vegetables and rely on servings of bread, rice, and pasta with every meal to help keep food moving through their digestive systems. These people may not be overweight at all—and may have tons of energy to burn during their daily exercise.

So, that's the point. Foods should no longer be looked at as good or bad—just about every food has both good and bad! Foods that are frequently considered "healthy" have unhealthy properties, and "unhealthy" foods have some healthy qualities. It is the balance of foods that is important. Too much or too little of any food or drink isn't good.

Take water, for instance! Too little water can lead to dehydration and death. Too much also has deadly consequences. Overhydration by athletes is called exercise-associated hyponatremia. It occurs when athletes drink even when they are not thirsty in an attempt to rehydrate, typically after endurance distances. Drinking too much during exercise can overwhelm the body's ability to remove water. The sodium content of blood is diluted to abnormally low levels. Cells absorb excess water, which can cause swelling—most dangerously in the brain.

Hyponatremia can cause muscle cramps, nausea, vomiting, seizures, unconsciousness, and, in rare cases, death. In 2007, a California woman died from water intoxication after drinking six liters of water—roughly twenty-five glasses—in three hours. In 2005, a fraternity hazing at California State University, Chico, left a twenty-one-year-old man dead after he was forced to drink excessive amounts of water between rounds of push-ups in a cold basement. Clubgoers taking MDMA ("ecstasy") have also died after consuming copious amounts of water trying to rehydrate following long nights of dancing and sweating.

So, what should you be eating and what should you be avoiding? Well, the answer is confusing! Here's why:

In her new book, *Unsavory Truth: How Food Companies Skew the Science of What We Eat*, Marion Nestle, an NYU professor in nutrition, food studies, and public health, shows how nutritional research is frequently funded and promoted by the food industry. Nestle writes, "Whenever I see a study suggesting that a single food (such as pork, oats, pears), eating pattern (having breakfast) or product (beef, diet sodas, chocolate) improves health, I look to see who paid for it," Nestle writes. "If an industry-funded study claims miraculous benefits from the sponsor's products, think: 'Advertising.'"

One of the most noteworthy research funders is Coca-Cola, which invested more than $6 million in a report called the International Study of Childhood Obesity, Lifestyle, and the Environment. It tracked 6,000 children, starting in 2010, and studied their physical activity, sleep, TV habits, and diet. Researchers did not include soda consumption in the study. They did find correlations between obesity and lack of sleep, low physical activity, and frequent TV watching. If Coca-Cola had included a question about soda, they likely would have found that the obese children studied were drinking soda—but that would damage their sales. "Coca-Cola could not have asked for a better outcome," Nestle writes.

This brings me back to thinking about diets and how they all seem to be successful. Diets rely on marketing. And all diets will only publicize the success stories. They also tend to reference certain cultures and societies or "science" to prove their point of lasting benefits. The raw food fad, for instance, points to our ancestors who didn't have modern cooking available and ate raw foods. The high-fat and protein supporters will cite cultures that consume large amounts of fat and live quite healthfully. The vegetarians study cultures that mainly subsist on rice and vegetables. These personal stories become a type of gospel in an effort to convince as many people as possible to join them. Books are then written on these diets, and entire industries are built around these beliefs, and those on the particular diet feel they are, indeed, "right." What is really right is what your body likes and thrives on, essentially what brings your individual body into balance.

THINK HARMONY AND BALANCE: YIN AND YANG

Extremes on either end are what creates the problem. When it comes to harmony in the body, too much of a good thing is just as bad as not enough. Too much roughage (too many raw fruits and vegetables, smoothies, and juices), for instance, often brings a health nut into my office complaining of reflexed back pain, and the gas and bloating from their diet is the root cause. Too much fast food and saturated fats for the on-the-go eater can cause weight gain and slow digestion.

Many different cultures describe the body in terms of energy or harmony and balance. Asian culture describes a yin and yang, a balance of two opposing forces. Indian culture follows an ayurvedic model of balancing pitta. No matter which specific belief you ascribe to, the concept of harmony and balance is vital, just in the way that the gas pedal and the brake in a car are both necessary, but at specific moments. In our Western culture, this approach of achieving balance seems to be missing. We tend to gravitate toward extremes, like binge diets. The harm in our foods is when we get stuck on a dogma and end up consuming too much or too little of one thing or food group. Salt, for instance, will raise sodium levels and elevate blood pressure if you take in too much; however, salt has been shown to have a great many medicinal properties and is necessary for our cellular makeup. Caffeine can act as a drug and stimulant and can become quite addictive, but caffeine has also proven to improve alertness and decrease headaches. We all know the dangers of too much alcohol, and yet there are many studies touting the benefits of a glass of red wine.

THE BODY NEEDS BALANCE

We should be thinking about food and drink in balance. The medical term for balance is *homeostasis*, which is defined as a relatively stable state of equilibrium or a tendency toward such a state between the different but interdependent elements of the body. The body is a self-regulating homeostatic balancing system that continually monitors and adjusts for many different conditions. Whether it's changing your blood flow, alertness, or heart rate, your body adjusts and adapts. Body temperature is a particularly easy-to-explain example of homeostasis. If you are too cold, your body will shiver to raise your body's temperature; if you are too hot, your body will perspire to cool down your body. Your body will either accomplish these things automatically or signal to you that you need to make some corrections (i.e., add or take off a layer of clothing). A good homeostatic state also applies to the digestive system: Your output is a language indicating balance or imbalance in your body and the expression of desire for different input as a means to regulate the stomach. I, in fact, thought about naming the book *The Homeostatic Diet*; however, it just wasn't as catchy as our current title!

THE GOOD SHIT DIET IS ALL BASED ON HAVING A GOOD SHIT

The right diet for you is the diet that produces homeostasis in your body. *The right diet for you is the diet that produces the right shit.* By the end of this book, you'll be on your way to balancing your input with your output and will begin understanding what homeostasis in your body actually feels like! Chances are, you are so well trained at ignoring your poop that you don't even know how poorly you are feeling!

2

Shit Happens!

How Your Shit Comes Together

From the moment food enters your mouth, your body begins to turn it into a soupy mush called *chyme*. Chewing, saliva, peristalsis (the involuntary contractions of gastrointestinal muscles), bacteria, hydrochloric acid, digestive enzymes, bile, and other secretions all work to break down your food. While your digestive cells absorb sugars, starches, fats, vitamins, minerals, and other nutrients, waste products continue traveling down the line. In the colon, all the leftovers are combined and packed together to form a stool. Stools consist mainly of water, mucous, indigestible fiber, old cells from your intestinal lining, millions of microorganisms (like living and dead bacteria), undigested food such as corn and small seeds, and small amounts of inorganic salts.

The time that food and drinks take to pass through your system is called its *transit time*. We need the proper transit time to ingest, digest, and excrete.

Transit times that are too quick don't allow the body to absorb all of the proper nutrients, and transit times that are too long allow bacteria and toxicity to build up in the body. It takes between three and ten hours for your large intestine to absorb enough water from waste material to turn it into solid or partially solid stools.

When your rectal pouch is distended with enough feces to trigger a contractile reflex, your feces are pushed out through your anus. When you consciously contract your abdominal wall, your diaphragm moves downward and helps open up muscles that line your anal sphincter. (Your rectum is lined with three horizontal folds, called your rectal valves, that prevent you from pooping when you fart! Thank you, rectum, for preventing the sharts.)

If all goes as it should, you'll end up with a healthy bowel movement, brown to light brown. (This color comes from the worn-out red blood cells in bile; formed but not hard; cylindrical, not flattened; fairly bulky and full-bodied, not compacted; somewhat textured but not too messy; and very easy to pass.) And it shouldn't smell—much. "You're passing methane and bacteria, degraded foodstuffs, so there's always going to be an odor," says Patrick Donovan, ND, a naturopath in Seattle. "But it shouldn't be a very strong, pungent odor."

WATCH YOUR SHIT!

Examining your shit is important to determine if your built-in detox system is working properly, and if you are indeed getting rid of your shit in a good way. The Bristol Stool Chart is a handy way to help you identify the shape, consistency, and color of your shit and determine if your insides are running efficiently. Types 3, 4, and 5 are the ideal poops, with Type 4 being optimum, and a sign that your body is in homeostasis and that you are putting the right foods into your body. After every shit, check it out to see what you created. Does it grade out to a perfect 4? If so, celebrate!

I bought myself a T-shirt that says, "I pooped today!" with quite a triumphant stick figure in celebration mode but, of course, my family won't let me wear it.

The Bristol Stool Form Scale

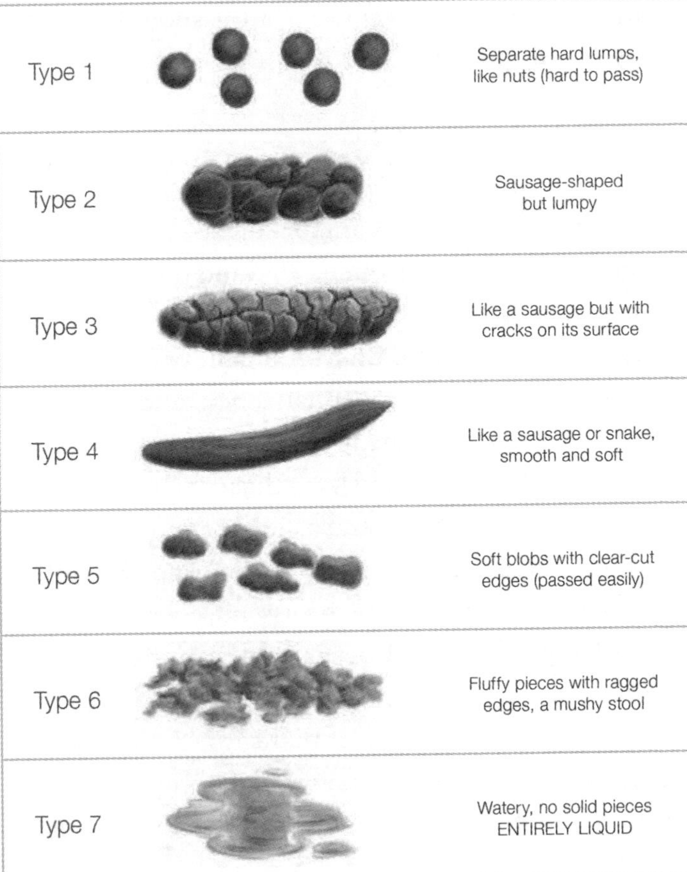

UK/COR/0118/0853. Date of preparation: January 2018

Shit Happens!

Now, you know what a good poop looks like. The second factor of a good shit is how often you have them!

WHY ARE REGULAR BOWEL MOVEMENTS SO IMPORTANT?

When we accept that our bowel movements are key predictors to our well-being and as useful in diagnosing our health as taking our temperature or our blood pressure, regularity takes on a lot more importance. When we talk about regularity, what we're really talking about is *what's regular for you.* If your shit is grading out to a 3 or 4, chances are that you are having the right regularity and frequency for you. Some people will poop three times a day while others go three times a week. As long as you are getting good grades and feel comfortable, you are in good shape.

Here are the top reasons why regularity is so important:

- **Toxin removal.** The bowel is the lower part of your digestive tract, which includes the small intestine, large intestine, and rectum. The functions of the bowel are to absorb nutrients and water from digested food, and to help the body form and excrete waste products in the form of stools. Your stools contain lots of toxins that need to be cleared regularly, otherwise the bowel will be the first part of your body to be affected. Bilirubin (a product of broken-down blood cells that gives the stool its brown color), for example, is one of the body's main toxic waste products excreted through the bowel.

- **Preventing illness.** Abnormal bowel movements can be a sign your diet isn't right for you, but they can also be symptoms of hemorrhoids, irritable bowel syndrome, Crohn's disease, ulcerative colitis, polyps, and bowel cancer. Regularity is associated with a lowered risk of developing any of these bowel issues.
- **Less bloat and more comfort.** Regular bowel movements allow for more efficient absorption of water and minerals, less gassiness,

and an overall feeling of lightness, comfort, and well-being in your abdominal region. This also leads to less muscular pain—specifically back and neck pain—which can be caused by irritation in the digestion system that reflexes into the back and radiates elsewhere.

LET YOUR SHIT SET YOU FREE

Patients will frequently ask about doing a cleanse or a detox or trying colonics. I tell them it's important that they realize their digestive and elimination system is a built-in detox system. I repeat: Bowel movements are your body's detox system. Simply put: If you are having good, healthy bowel movements, then your body is ridding yourself of your waste products properly and you should not need a separate cleansing. I do know patients, however, who have had great relief from colonics. My recommendation is to use them as a last resort after you have tried to balance both the output and the input aspects of your digestive system. Colonics are great to clean you out, but, ideally, you want to identify the cause of the imbalance and avoid having to use them. If you are irregular or having bad poops, one cleanse is not going to change things for you if you continue eating in a way that's causing imbalance!

Probiotics are used more widely than colonics. They promise to help your digestive system get and stay on track, but probiotics work much in the same way as food—sometimes they are healthy for people, sometimes they are not! I have seen instances where they can be the cure of back pain—or the cause!

I'd like to tell you a story of a patient of mine named Rob Ernst, who is in his early forties and married with three kids. Rob leads quite an active lifestyle and travels extensively for work. One day, he came to me complaining of mid-back pain that just didn't seem to be going away. After treating him structurally for a few weeks with manipulation, massage, heat, electrical stimulation, and stretches, the pain was still there. I therefore turned my attention to other factors: Could it be his stress? He claimed that he felt pretty relaxed and that everything was really going great. I asked about his diet, and he said not much had changed since the onset of his pain, except that a few weeks ago, his wife saw a television show on the power of probiotics and started to give him one to take every morning. He went on to say that the probiotic seemed to throw off his stomach a bit and gave him a bit of gas, but he kept taking it because it was supposed to be good for him. I told him what he said made sense, but if the probiotic was upsetting his stomach, it might not be helping him. I recommended that he stop taking the probiotic for two weeks and see how he felt. Not only did the gas go away, but the back pain did as well. The cause of Rob's back pain was actually his probiotic!

Conversely, I had a patient who was suffering from both lower back pain and an upset stomach but who ate a wide variety of noninflammatory foods. Willow Jarosh, an expert nutritionist, recommended a probiotic to help balance my patient's stomach. Two weeks after taking the probiotic, my patient's stomach was calmed down, and her pain was much improved!

Every body is different. A probiotic is input; it may help you and it may not! The goal of this book is to give you a gut that works optimally as your built-in detox system. If you are still struggling even though your input is ultimately balanced, you might need the support of a probiotic.

3

That's Some Bad Shit!

After reviewing the Bristol Stool Chart, you may be realizing that your poop typically does *not* fall into healthy Types 3 or 4.

WHAT ARE SOME OTHER INDICATORS OF AN UNHEALTHY BOWEL MOVEMENT?

- Bowel movements with very hard, loose, smelly, or sticky stools (so Types 1 and 6 on the chart, especially)
- Bowel movements with abdominal pain or blood in the stool
- Infrequent (typically less than daily) or irregular bowel movements
- Sluggish bowel movements that are difficult to pass and don't feel complete afterward
- Abdominal bloating and passing lots of smelly wind

- Hemorrhoids: pain or burning sensation around the anus
- Very pale or very dark stools

BODY SYMPTOMS FROM AN UNHEALTHY BOWEL

When too many toxins build up in the bowel, this can affect the whole body and cause other symptoms such as:

- Tired, heavy, and puffy body
- Headache
- Insomnia, vivid dreams
- Lower back pain
- Red face and red nose
- Skin rashes
- Bad breath
- Weight gain

If you are experiencing stools that are not Type 3 and 4, and are regularly experiencing Types 1 or 6, as well as any of the symptoms indicated above, you are having some really bad shits. Here is another handy poop chart (adapted from PreventDisease.com) that further explains the appearance of bad stools and what they could mean about your health.

IF YOUR STOOL LOOKS LIKE . . .	IT COULD MEAN . . .
Black, tarry, and sticky	Bleeding in your upper digestive tract. The black color comes from digested blood cells.
Very dark brown	You drank red wine last night or have too much salt or not enough vegetables in your diet.
Glowing red or magenta	You've eaten a lot of reddish foods, such as beets.
Light green	You're consuming too much sugar or too many fruits and vegetables with not enough grains or salt.

The Good Shit

IF YOUR STOOL LOOKS LIKE . . .	IT COULD MEAN . . .
Pale or clay-colored	Minimal amounts of bile are being excreted, perhaps because of problems with the gallbladder or liver.
Bloody or mucus-covered	Hemorrhoids, an overgrowth of certain bacteria in your gastrointestinal tract, colitis (inflammation of the colon), Crohn's disease (also known as inflammatory bowel disease), or colon cancer. Red blood usually means the ailment is located near the end of your digestive tract, whereas black blood signals partially digested blood coming from an ailment higher up the tract. Seek medical advice promptly.

That's Some Bad Shit!

IF YOUR STOOL LOOKS LIKE . . .	IT COULD MEAN . . .
Pencil-thin and ribbonlike	A polyp or growth in your colon that narrows the passage for stool.
Large and floating, with greasy film on toilet water	Malabsorption—your digestive system isn't getting the full nutritional use of food.
Loose and watery, sometimes with undigested foodstuffs	Diarrhea. Possible causes are food poisoning, lactose intolerance, antibiotics, antacids, dietary changes, travel, anxiety, stress, inflammatory bowel disease, or irritable bowel syndrome.
Small, hard, round pellets	Constipation—even if you're defecating frequently. Possible causes are: eating too much dry food, including protein, and not enough vegetables and raw foods; laxative abuse; worries; or irritable bowel syndrome.

The most common types of these bad shits are those associated with diarrhea and constipation. Why do diarrhea and constipation happen?

DIARRHEA EXPLAINED

When waste material travels through your digestive tract too quickly for sufficient water absorption to occur, your stools will be runny and more frequent than normal.

Three main causes of diarrhea are:

- Undesirable microorganisms
- Food intolerances (like lactose intolerance)
- Stress

In the first two cases, it makes sense that your body would want things to move quickly through your system: Your body doesn't want to spend time digesting foods that it can't properly extract nutrients from or that are laced with disease-causing microbes. Food intolerance may not even mean you have a diagnosable problem, like celiac disease. It might be as simple as my own discovery—big salads make me prone to diarrhea! My stomach just doesn't tolerate them as nicely as a sandwich. This is where you may need to tune in to your own body language and not ignore the signs it is sending you!

Stress can cause the shits! This is because stress shortens the transit time by messing with your enteric nervous system (the part that regulates your physiological responses to emotional and physical stress).

CONSTIPATION EXPLAINED

Here's a bad—but true—constipation joke: People who are constipated couldn't give a shit!

Now really, constipation can be uncomfortable! When waste material travels through your colon more slowly than it should, enough water is extracted from your waste material to cause your stools to become uncomfortably hard. You may find that they are also pellet-like, as shown in Type 1 of The Bristol Stool Chart.

Five main causes of constipation are:

- Eating sporadically or eating meals that are too small to elicit mass peristalsis.
- Not going when you feel an urge to go.
- Lack of a healthy intestinal lining that is capable of producing enough mucous to properly lubricate your stools (vitamin A deficiency is a potential cause of this situation).
- Insufficient intake of water, water-rich foods, or fiber-rich foods.
- Stress (yes, it doesn't just cause the runs!).

GAS EXPLAINED

Digestive dysfunction and problems with the ileocecal valve can create gas. Gas sounds a bit stinky but may not seem like a big deal. Yet it is! Excessive or stinky gas is a sign that your body does not like the foods it's digesting. Back pain can also sometimes be caused by excess gas in your gut. The trapped gas and bloating caused by digestive irritation creates swelling in the abdomen, putting pressure on the back and spine and resulting in lower or middle back pain. If these two symptoms seem to occur in tandem, your bloating may be giving rise to your lower back pain.

Here is an example of an X-ray that exhibits a healthy stomach:

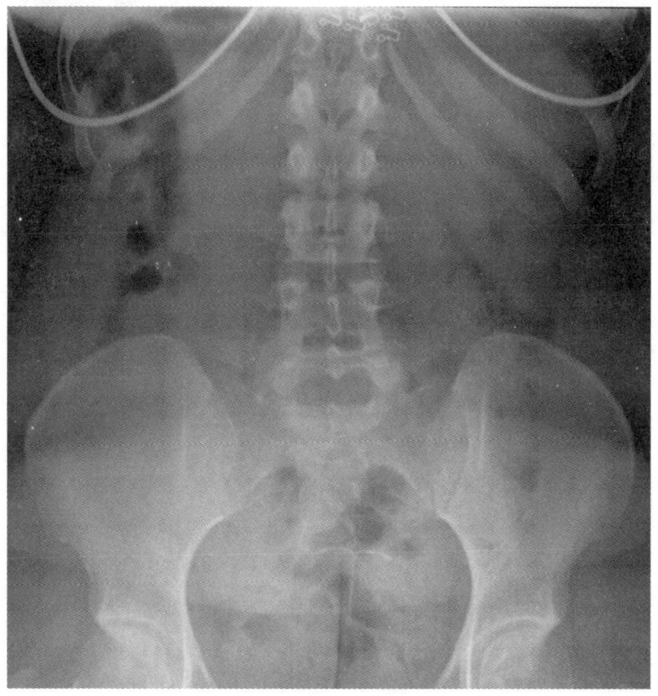

Healthy Stomach

You'll see there is a clear image of the spine and pelvic bones.

Now, compare this to the X-rays of two people with substantial gas!

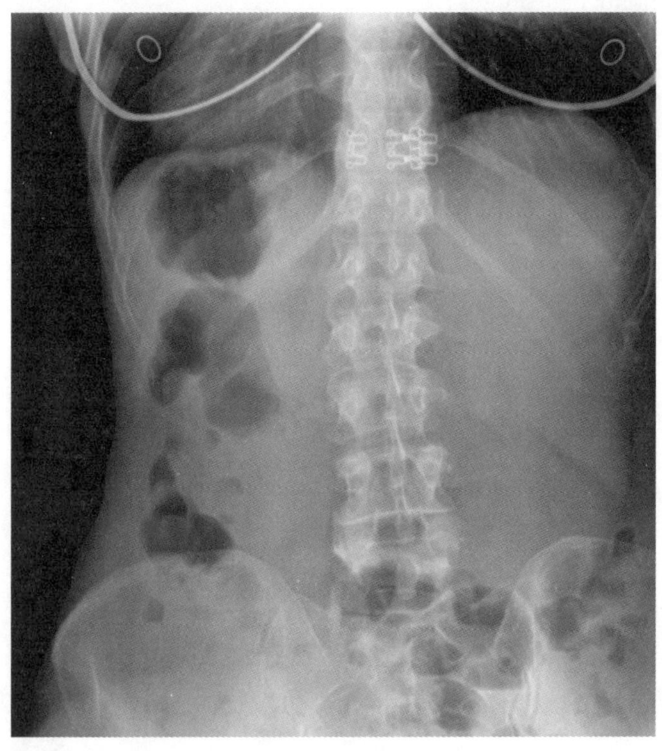

Moderate Gas

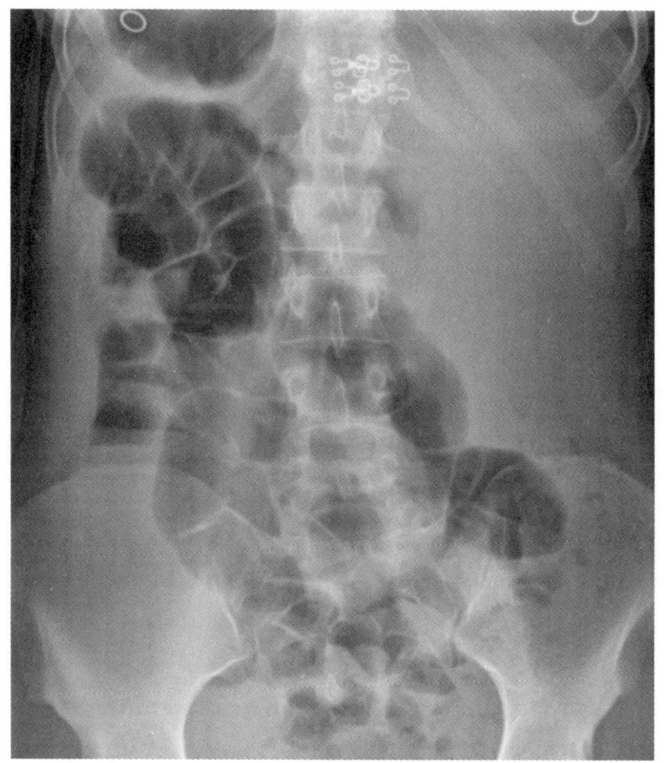

Heavy Gas

Do you see all the circles, or gas bubbles, throughout the abdomen? The first X-ray (on page 50) reveals moderate gas. In the X-ray on this page, there is so much gas that you can't get a good look at the patient's bones. But you certainly can see what is causing their discomfort! For gas to show up on an X-ray like this, there has to be about fourteen pounds of gas per square inch! For comparison's sake, a football (no Tom Brady jokes!) has about thirteen-and-a-half pounds of gas per square inch, while a basketball has seven-and a-half pounds of gas per square inch. People are frequently walking around with gas pressure in their abdominal cavity that is equal to the pressure of an inflated football and don't even know it! They tend to think that it's normal because they are used to feeling that way. They may not even consider themselves "gassy" people, because the gas just gets trapped in the stomach and doesn't pass frequently. Interestingly enough, these people come to me complaining of back pain, not abdominal pain. Once you see this on an X-ray, however, you know that reducing the gas and inflammation in the gut is vital to ridding the patient of the back pain. Frequently, patients will only realize how uncomfortable they were digestively after a diet change eliminates the gas and bloating.

That's Some Bad Shit!

For me, the frustrating part is that radiologists will disregard these very clear X-ray findings, because they are trained to look only for fractures, tumors, diseases, and arthritis. That is why many doctors aren't diagnosing you correctly and are missing the diet connection completely!

DIAGNOSING BOWEL PROBLEMS

If you are suffering from irregularity, stomach pain, constipation, diarrhea, or other bowel-related issues, I recommend keeping a record for a week to ten days and then sharing it with a health practitioner. In addition to telling your doctor your diet history, if you are prone to hemorrhoids or have had any diseases of the rectum, and both current and previous medication/laxative use, you should record the following for each bowel movement:

- What does the stool look like? What is the color, shape, and texture? (Use the two poop charts to help you describe each bowel movement!)

- Did you have to strain to defecate?
- Did you soil your underwear before making it to the toilet?
- Did you have any pain in the rectum, or any stomach pain? Is this pain related to defecation?
- Was there any blood or mucous in your stool?
- Are you stressed?
- Did you exercise today? If you are training, are you noticing other overtraining symptoms, like muscle aches or fatigue? How do you feel during and in between workouts and how do you feel after taking a day off?

This last question goes back to the idea of homeostasis. Poop usually improves when your body hits the right balance: some exercise, not too much. Keeping track of how you feel when exercising will help you arrive at the right amount for your body.

All these points together, as well as your digestive history, are important in determining how best to manage the problems you are having, and to decide whether you need any tests to eliminate the possibility of serious bowel disease. It's especially important to make sure you don't forget to give your doctor a list of all your medications. Medications are a serious culprit of bowel problems. Antihypertensive drugs, calcium channel-blockers, and anticonvulsants may present problems. Iron and calcium supplements—both of which may be very important as supplemental nutrients in the elderly—and aluminum containing antacid compounds may cause constipation. Also, drugs that are used for the treatment of Parkinson's disease, antidepressants, and antipsychotic medications are all common causes of bowel roadblocks.

4

Get Your Shit Checked

The Importance of the Colonoscopy and Early Detection of Colorectal Cancer

MY COLONOSCOPY EXPERIENCE

I had the unfortunate pleasure of meeting Dr. Procaccino in 2018 after my mom was diagnosed with colon cancer and it was discovered that there were three tumors that needed to be removed surgically. After meeting Dr. Procaccino, my mom, sister, and I knew we had found the right surgeon: He was the perfect match of clinical skills and just the right bedside manner. After a surgery and subsequent second surgery to correct Mom's temporary ostomy bag, I came to the realization that I now had a family history of colon cancer. At forty-nine years old, it was time for my first colonoscopy and there was no doubt who would do it: Dr. Procaccino!

When I told my friends that I had scheduled my colonoscopy, they all snickered and said, "*That* will be an interesting process!" I agreed, imagining the preparation day and how I would have to drink maybe five gallons of literally undrinkable fluid and then be stuck in the bathroom for hours with uncontrollable diarrhea. I can tell you, without out a doubt, that the hype was way worse than the process. In reality, I had to drink a dose of medicine that was slightly larger than the size of a double shot of alcohol followed by five glasses of liquid over the next three hours. I repeated the process. The liquids I was allowed had to be clear, avoiding certain dyes. For instance, you can drink lemon Gatorade or even have lime Jell-O but cannot ingest red dye. I had miso soup, chicken broth, water, clear apple juice, and lemon Italian ice.

Now let's discuss the diarrhea. It was bad, I won't lie. Never have I had the feeling of literally peeing out of my ass that I had with this process. This wasn't my favorite part, but it wasn't as horrifically awful as I had expected. I felt empty and light, which was quite a pleasant surprise.

The next morning, I went to the appointment with some apprehension. After signing the scary waiver forms, I was given some medication that evidently put me into a deep slumber. Next thing I knew, I was awakening from a great nap quite hungry! The entire procedure, from the time I entered the office to leaving, took an hour. Thankfully, everything checked out just fine for me, and I will need to do this again in five years because of my family history. This colonoscopy really wasn't bad at all, and I urge people not to be scared of it! Besides, you can really treat yourself after! My post-procedure meal of strawberry pancakes washed down with chocolate milk at IHOP was quite yummy!

ASK DOCTOR PROCACCINO

I really wanted to dive into the recent changes in colonoscopy guidelines as part of this chapter, so I went right to the expert and interviewed my own GI doctor, John Procaccino, a colorectal surgeon on Long Island. Here are my burning colon questions for him and his convincing answers.

Question: Colorectal cancer has been on the rise in recent years. Can you explain the causes of colon cancer and the theory of colonoscopy as a preventative, not just a diagnostic, treatment?

Dr. Procaccino: In America, the number-one killer is now cancer. It used to be cardiovascular disease, but recently, they flip-flopped. Of the cancers that kill us, the most frequent killer is lung cancer, directly correlated with smoking. The second most common cause of cancer death is colorectal cancer in both sexes, which is very significant. Ninety-five percent of colon and rectal cancer is sporadic, meaning there's not a family history involved. There are genetically linked syndromes (for example, Lynch Syndrome, Familial Polyposis, etc.), but the vast majority are what we call sporadic. And the vast majority of the time, these sporadic cancers arise from a benign precursor stage called a polyp. Now it can take from two to six years to go from nothing to a polyp to a cancer. Not every polyp is going to become a cancer, but almost every cancer came from what was once a polyp. The vast majority of these polyps are asymptomatic, so the theory behind colonoscopy is the following: If you are colonoscoped, and if a polyp is seen and removed, the analogy that I use is it's like taking dandelions out of your lawn in the spring before they go to seed and overrun the lawn.

Colonoscopy

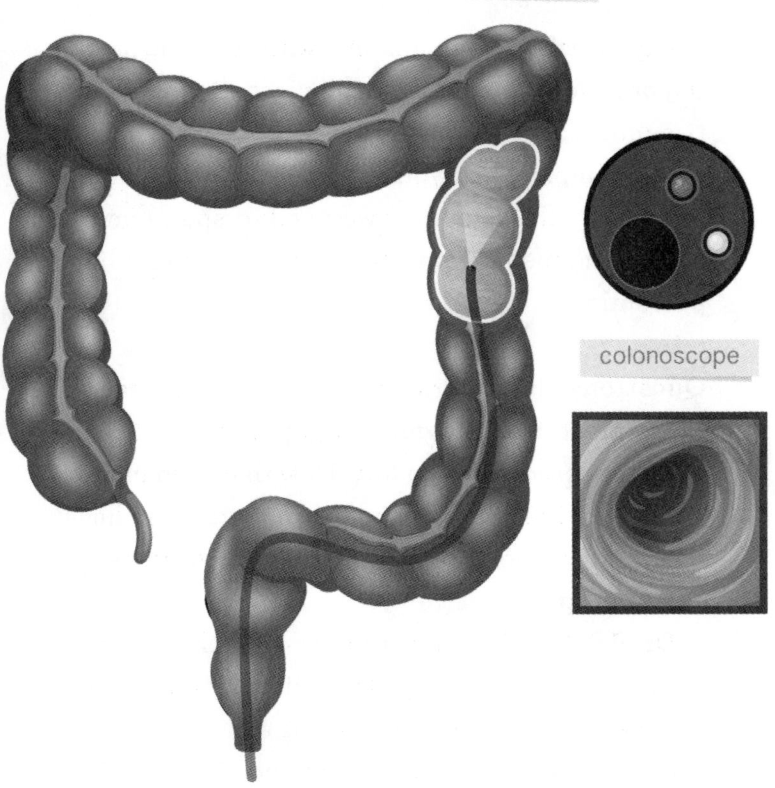

If you eat a balanced diet and get a colonoscopy, you are almost going to eliminate the second most common cause of cancer death in the U.S., which is pretty amazing. If you link that with stopping smoking or never smoking, again you just eliminated the two most common causes of cancer death, which is pretty simple when you consider people freaking out about all this money we need to spend on research and medications. But that's the bottom line: prevention.

Question: The American Cancer Society used to recommend that the general population get their first colonoscopy at age fifty. Now that is changing, and the guidelines are suggesting everyone have their first colonoscopy at age forty-five. Why the decrease in age?

Dr. P.: One of the most interesting changes I've seen in the epidemiology of this disease is that when I trained thirty years ago, this was a disease of people in their sixties and seventies and eighties. With every passing year, we are seeing cancer more commonly in people in their twenties, thirties, and forties. We don't have the answer yet as to why. One of the theories is disruption of the microbiome. Within our colon live zillions of bacteria, which have a protective effect. So, we're just not quite sure why or what's changing this biome and if that is, in fact, a potential causative agent. Could it be related to processed foods, antibiotics, something that we're putting into our body? We don't know. But it's a hot topic, and I think it's got to be related [to a change in our input], when you think of things that have changed over the last thirty years.

Another amazing postulate is this: There's theoretically stuff in our waste that would have a negative effect on the colonic cells. The lining of the colon is made of these cells, which look like the pink glistening lining cells inside your mouth. They're called mucosa because they produce mucous, a slippery substance to let things go through. The theory is if there is something sitting in contact with the colonic cells longer, maybe that triggers an abnormal response of these cells turning over. So, one of the theories that was purported by this guy who gave a lecture [at a conference I just went to] was,

"What's changed over the last thirty years?" Well, younger people don't go out and do physical activity. They sit and they play video games for hours at a clip. The place where stool is stored normally is in the left colon, the sigmoid colon, and it only comes into the rectum when a fill point is reached. A vast majority of cancers we are seeing in the younger population is in that location. So, his theory is kids are putting off having bowel movements while they are sitting around playing these games and maybe that is causing this. I mean, it's bizarre, but it's as good as any other explanation!

Question: So the increase of cancer in younger people resulted in the decrease of age in colonoscopy guidelines?

Dr. P.: Yes. It's got a great effect because the guidelines that exist on screening are determined by big organizations: The American Cancer Society, The American Society of Colorectal Surgeons, The American College of Gastroenterologists. Older studies show the instances of polyps went up over the age of fifty, and cancer went up a few years after that based on the polyp sequence I told you about. So, when you look at graphs of age distribution and numbers of cancers as they are going up with each decade of life and also with each decade that passes, we are seeing a decrease in colon cancer instances in older age groups. The only explanation for that is increased screening and removal of polyps at the other end of that.

[Screening younger is] a very, very important topic to me because in the last month I operated on a thirty-seven-year-old woman and a forty-six-year-old man. It seems to be the [younger you see them, the more aggressive they get]. Or they are further along in the staging because bleeding is often attributed to hemorrhoids or God knows what because it isn't [the inclination] to do a colonoscopy on a thirty-seven-year-old.

Question: How is a patient with family history treated differently in terms of age for their first colonoscopy?

Dr. P.: The guidelines backed off from fifty, now down to forty-five—that's with negative family history. If a first-degree relative (i.e., mother, father, sibling) has been diagnosed with a colorectal cancer, they are supposed to be scoped at the latest ten years before normal. Instead of fifty, it's forty, perhaps even thirty-five. Why? Because the incidence of colorectal cancer in the first-degree relatives of those who have it is three to ten times greater than the general population. Specimens are [now] being sent out for certain genetic testing to see if it falls into that 5 percent of genetically linked or family cancer syndromes. Why is that so important? Because you would really start screening earlier and more frequently, and those individuals often have multi-cancer syndromes, where there's a genetic link to gynecological cancers, malignancy, thyroid, colon, bladder, etc., so it's critical to make sure you don't have that.

Question: And what about frequency of colonoscopies with a family history?

Dr. P.: That depends upon when the earliest member of the family had it. If you get a baseline scope and it's negative, you don't need another one for five years. If it's scoped and you have a polyp, you should have another one in three years, unless it's what we call a high-risk polyp, which would be something with dysplasia, or pre-cancer cells, in it, and those may be rescoped in a year. The interval is contingent upon what the findings are and, if there is a polyp, what the histologic final diagnosis is.

Question: I'm telling my readers about the colonoscopy prep and how it isn't as bad as all that. What do you have to say about the prep process?

Dr. P.: What you're taking now is much better. What we used to have was Go Lightly, which was very large volume, oily in consistency, very difficult to get down. It's almost like every year, another prep comes out. The volume now is lower and more palatable.

The way I look at it is this: Having diarrhea for three hours and taking a bowel prep, which can potentially save your life, you can't complain about it and say, "I'm not going to get a colonoscopy because I don't want to take that prep." It just doesn't flow with me. Plus, it's an absolutely painless procedure.

It's less uncomfortable than a woman going to the gynecologist or a man having his prostate checked because you are sedated. You don't even know anything happened. You close your eyes and you open them and the procedure is over.

People say, well there's a very high complication rate. Well, you know what, the risk of major complication is between 1 in 2,000 and 1 in 4,000 in the hands of a Board Certified individual who's given the privilege of doing this. The rate of a polyp is 1 in 5 and the rate of a cancer is 1 in 17. Just play simple odds. Is there anything you do in life that has no risk? Getting in your car and driving to work, getting on an airplane, going down to New York City. What I'm trying to say is: Be in touch with your own body and take responsibility for your own health. It's not the government's job; it's not your doctor's total job to take care of you. You have to present yourself to the doctor. You know how many people say to me, "I never knew I had a problem. I never had a colonoscopy"? I ask, "When did you last see a doctor?" They say, "Well, I had no problems so I didn't go to the doctor." That's like saying to me, "I didn't bring my car to get my transmission fluid changed after 100,000 miles and now he tells me I need a new transmission, can you believe that?" It's preventative maintenance. That's what this is. Preventative maintenance. Life is precious. It is a beautiful gift and we can live longer because we have all this technology.

Question: I've heard about the Cologuard screening, which uses your stools to detect cancer or precancer. Is it a good screen?

Dr. P.: It doesn't replace a colonoscopy, but it is much better than the old-time guaiac or fecal occult blood testing. That was a hydrogen peroxidous reaction, and [it had] a high degree of false negatives and false positives. You ate meat in the last week and that could falsely make it positive. So, it was almost like a coin toss. It came up to be about 30 to 50 percent inaccurate. Cologuard is a test that is based on antigens on the surface of tumor cells that are shed into the stool and it's pretty darn accurate for saying if you have colon cancer. Your doctor has to order it because it's costly, and you bring it home and you put your waste matter in this reaction thing and you send it off. I'm not quite sure when it should start, but I think with what we are seeing now, it's valid to start doing it over the age of thirty.

Question: Speaking of studying stool, why are regular bowel movements so important?

Dr. P.: More than anything, it's an indication of overall body health. It's something that's very overt and obvious and you can track it. Again, there's the theory, if you are not having regular bowel movements, maybe the stuff that's remaining in your colon, the waste products of what you're eating, could have some sort of a toxic or negative effect because it's staying in contact with the normal lining of your rectum for longer periods of time. It's soft, but it's a theory that exists. Now, there are other conditions that increase one's risk of developing colorectal cancer. Examples are inflammatory conditions such as inflammatory bowel disease, Crohn's disease and ulcerative colitis. Now, these cause inflammation and therefore more activity of the colonic lining cells and certainly increase one's risk.

Question: What questions do you ask patients about their bowel movements?

Dr. P.: The human body generally lives in a state of homeostasis, [meaning] things are very normal on a day-to-day basis. Most people in this country have breakfast, have a cup of coffee, and have a bowel movement after that. That's the vast majority of the way people's intestinal tracks work. Asking one about a change in bowel habits is critical because often that's the first harbinger of a potential problem. If a growth is developing in the colon and the internal diameter of the colon is changing, then what can get past it changes. That doesn't mean you have to be constipated. Sometimes going more frequently is a sign of a potential issue because only smaller amounts of waste are getting past this problem. This [example] pertains to lesions that are on the left side of your colon. What does that mean? The colon is five feet in length and is a waste processing plant, meaning it takes high-volume liquid stool on the right, and as it traverses that five-foot pipe, the lining takes the fluid out of it and changes it to low-volume solid. The point is that lesions on the right side of the colon can hide there a lot longer before they become symptomatic because liquid can pass big things for a long time before you know about it, as opposed to the left side where the stool is solid, so it's not the greatest [means of detection] for all cancers of the colon. But a change is critical. Any blood in your bowel movements needs to be investigated. And there are questions. Is it bright red? Is it painless? Is it seen on wiping or dripping in the bowl? These are more indicative of hemorrhoidal bleeding. Stool with blood in it is a flashing red light. Weight loss, change in appetite, new onset abdominal pain. These are often later on the continuum of the disease entity. The vast majority of patients with colon cancer have no symptoms. It's a silent killer. But it is a highly preventable cancer by doing what we said.

Question: Is there a normal frequency of bowel movements that indicates to you optimal colon health?

Dr. P.: General rule of thumb, the way the human body works, is that in a twenty-four hour period, there is normally a need to clear the bowels once a day. That would be general on a bell curve. There are people on either end of that, and it doesn't necessarily indicate pathology. But when one has their intestinal tract functioning in a certain way forever and then it changes, that's the biggest potential flashing red light.

Question: Someone told me about a fecal transplant. What is that about?

Dr. P.: That's mainly been used for a condition called C. diff, or Clostridium Difficil, which is an overgrowth of a toxic bacterium in the colon. The most common cause of C. diff is taking antibiotics exogenously. It can disrupt the balance of the microbiome, causing an overgrowth of C. diff. We see it in hospital settings because a lot of people are on antibiotics and it can be transmitted very easily from one patient to another, which is why terminal cleaning of the rooms is very important when the room changes and why the hospital staff is supposed to wash their hands between patient encounters. But C. diff is rampant. It comes with a 15 to 20 percent recurrence rate after initial treatment. Ironically, the treatment for it is another antibiotic. And once you've had one recurrence, the chance of having another recurrence is 50 percent. Some people get refractory C. diff, which can sometimes cause you such illness that the only way to survive is to have your whole colon removed, which can result in a permanent bag in your side.

But lately, what's been done is these fecal transplants, which try to restore the normal flora back in one's colon. Nowadays, the vast majority of time, that's instilled into the colon via a colonoscope. I just heard at this conference where they're trying, believe it or not, to develop some attenuated bacteria that you can take orally to perhaps reestablish this, which is a much easier way. It definitely has promise, it has great data to support it, and will be used frequently for these refractory cases.

Question: Do you have opinions on laxative or antacid use or current diet trends?

Dr. P.: I believe anything that's balanced is good. Whenever you live in one extreme or the other, it's a potential issue. Anything done to excess just doesn't work right. Drinking is okay, but drinking five drinks a day is not okay. Running twenty miles a day might not be the smartest thing for you. I don't think you shouldn't eat red meat. I don't think you should eat red meat six days in a row, though.

Question: How important is it to examine your own shit?

Dr. P.: How else would you know if you were having bleeding, unless you bleed to the point of soaking through your undergarments! If you just stand up, and you clean yourself and flush the bowl without looking back, [you'll never know]. It's like a woman examining her own breast. The easiest way to find a breast cancer that's not a microscopic cancer is for an individual to examine themselves. Who knows their body more than you?

GOT IT, DOC!

The two takeaways that I learned were:

1. Colorectal cancer is just about entirely preventable.
2. Three hours of diarrhea can save your life.

If this doesn't convince you to schedule your colonoscopy, I'm not sure what will!

5

Stress Screws Shit Up

Take stress seriously. Think about how to take care of you. (You're worth it, after all.)

Have you heard the phrase "I am so nervous, I am shitting in my pants"? This is not just a meaningless phrase. The impact emotions and stress have on your digestive system and shits is well documented. Stress or nervous stomach causes the release of hormones and neurotransmitters in the intestines and will frequently lead to loose stools (that is, "the shits"). On the flip side, others hold stress in their stomach, clenching their stomach muscles and their butt cheeks, thereby keeping everything in for too long and causing constipation.

Most people identify their biggest stressors as work and finances, or life events, like moving or a breakup. One of the things that people forget to equate with stress is grief. I experienced this firsthand. Right after my father passed away, I had a lot of stomach pain after drinking orange juice. When I was in a state of acute grief, I just couldn't digest all that acid. It wasn't until a year later that I could finally drink orange juice in the morning without it bothering me. This was a stress-induced digestive issue. I really had to listen to the language of my body, as well as align the issue with what was happening in my life to understand the correlation.

EMOTIONAL EATING

The link between emotions and eating has been well publicized, but, in my opinion, is misunder-stood. The connection goes much deeper than "emotional eating." Your emotional state when consuming a meal or a snack dramatically determines your digestive process. Here's an example: If you are eating a hot fudge sundae when you are depressed, there is a completely different biochemical process than if you are having the sundae as part of a celebration. Your body produces different neuropeptides and hormones in a state of depression than it does in a state of happiness, and this affects how your metabolism functions. It also explains why people could go wildly off their normally regimented diet on vacation and feel great; however, if they did that in their normal environment, they would suffer terribly. This also explains how one person might eat very little and not lose weight, while another person might take in more calories and seem not to gain weight.

If you are finding yourself suddenly in a similar position, ask yourself, "Am I eating with regret or joy?" "Am I feeling differently after consuming certain foods during times of stress?"

Simply put, a healthy relationship with eating is vital to being healthy, and a food that's healthy for you at one point in time may not be so good for you at another!

MY SUPERFOOD: Birthday Cake

If you were to ask me my recommendation for the best superfood, it would be birthday cake. For the most part, everyone likes their birthday. It is a time when friends and family get together to celebrate that they existed on this earth for another 365 days. This celebration even comes with presents, and who doesn't like presents? When we are eating birthday cake, our immune system is functioning at its peak because of our happiness. Our body produces neuropeptides and hormones during moments of joy that allow it to have the most efficient digestive process.

Most people equate emotional eating with eating junk food, but it's also important to acknowledge the emotional quotient if you are eating foods that are supposedly healthy but you are hating every moment of it. Is it then really "healthy"? Enjoying food/eating food you consider delicious is super important to so many aspects of overall health!

FOOD AND POOP CULTURE

This discussion of digestion and emotions leads me to something scientists and authors have studied for a long time: a look at other cultures to see what correlation diets have on longevity. The Mediterranean diet has received accolades for being the healthiest of diets filled with fish, healthy oils, and vegetables; however, there has been some evidence as of late that refutes that claim. A French diet, for instance, consists of large amounts of fats, dairy, and wine; and the French tend to have similar longevity. This dichotomy has left researchers quite bewildered. However, this makes perfect sense to me because the researchers only tend to look at foods and not the culture around the foods. I believe that the timing of the meals, the portion sizes, the quality of the ingredients as well as the emotional feeling around food will impact health and longevity as much as a particular food will.

So, how is the French diet similar to the Mediterranean diet? The food may not be similar, but the emotional environment *around* the food is similar. Both cultures sit down for meals—they do not eat on the go, they do not snack, and meals are treated as a time to gather and enjoy. Perhaps the areas of the world that seem to be living longer are happier and celebrate their meals, rather than stress eating! When meals are consumed in a leisurely way and the food is enjoyed, the result can be some really great shits!

LISTEN TO YOUR BODY

The First Step in Combating Emotional Eating

Just because your taste buds like something doesn't mean your stomach does. Your body knows what is good for it and what isn't; you just have to listen and obey. If you had Chinese food last night and you don't feel well this morning, ask yourself whether it was the three beers you had with dinner or the food itself. If you routinely get a stomachache after consuming milk products, you might have lactose intolerance. If you really pay attention to your body's signals, you can avoid the things that upset your system and find relief in both your stomach and your back!

Did Your "Healthful" Choice Satisfy?

I often find that those low-fat, "healthy" labels can make you overeat—big-time. For my patients experimenting with low-fat options like fat-free salad dressing or "healthy" substitutions like gluten-free bread and almond milk yogurt, they feel less satisfied and need more of the food to feel content with their meal, resulting in higher calorie consumption. I myself have found that I eat more when trying to choose a "healthier" substitute. I used to eat fruit-flavored cookies with the thought that I was eating a healthy version but would sometimes have more cookies in the end because I wasn't satisfied. So, which is better: two Oreos or four fruit cookies?

Many low-fat or fat-free foods use chemicals to simulate a flavor, so it's no wonder many of my patients complaining of digestive issues or gut-related back pain have recently started a new diet and are experiencing problems from it! In a 2015 study titled "The Effect of Fitness Branding on Restrained Eaters' Food Consumption and Post-Consumption Physical Activity," coauthors Hans Baumgartner(of Penn State) and Joerg Koenigstorfer (of Technische Universität München in Munich, Germany) found that the more fitness-branded foods dieters bought, the more they ate, and the less they exercised. I have seen this happen as well—when people think they are eating better, they feel they can exercise less. All of these effects are more negative than the effects of your previous, supposedly "unhealthy," diet!

Food or Therapy?

Food is meant to be eaten. Emotions are meant to be handled. Your emotional state and relationship with food need to be mutually supportive in order to regulate your digestive process. Not paying attention to this relationship is why many people end up with digestively induced back pain, weight gain from emotional eating, and other food-related issues. Sometimes, it's just about becoming more mindful of your body and its messages. Sometimes, issues with foods are much bigger. If this feels to be the case with you, a therapist might be helpful in starting this process.

A PATIENT STORY (SARAH LAFONTAINE)

Throughout college and grad school, I had a lot of stomach issues. I would eat something and swell up. I wasn't just getting bloated; I was constantly feeling sick and in pain.

I knew my body was inflamed, and I knew I had a family history (my mom had also struggled with lifelong stomach issues and ultimately was diagnosed with colitis), but I just didn't want to deal with it. Eventually, my mom went gluten-free and found a lot of relief for her colitis. Because I thought I had issues similar to hers, I decided to go completely gluten-free and to try and avoid dairy myself. Over the next six months, I gained eleven pounds and didn't find any relief from my pain and puffiness. It only got worse. Finally, at age twenty-five, I went to a gastroenterologist. When my blood test for allergies came up negative, the doctor felt I should get a colonoscopy. My mother and I both felt I was too young and was sure diet and nutrition was my problem. But this doctor made me paranoid, so I did both a colonoscopy and an endoscopy. When she called with the results, she said the endoscopy showed acid reflux, and the colonoscopy showed that my colon was "damaged." She suggested ulcerative colitis was likely or that there was possible scarring from too much pain medication (from ibuprofen) or from a previous virus or infection. I sobbed, thinking there was something really wrong with me. I decided to get a second opinion. I brought the results of my colonoscopy to a different doctor, who said that not only was my colon not damaged, but it was totally normal. This doctor felt I had IBS, which was more in line with what I had been feeling when I first sought help. But now, I was confused and upset. I didn't know what to do.

Meanwhile, my parents had been seeing Dr. Sinett and raved about him. I was hesitant, because I thought chiropractors were just a quick fix. But my parents were insistent that Dr. Sinett could help me with everything—even my stress and anxiety, which seemed to be exacerbating my stomach distress. My dad made an appointment for me. I told Dr. Sinett about my gluten-free diet and subsequent weight gain and explained how uncomfortable, swollen, and puffy I felt. I also had developed lower back pain in recent months, along with a worsening of the plantar fasciitis in my feet. Dr. Sinett did a physical check and saw that I had an imbalance in my feet, but he also did X-rays and saw a lot of gas. He felt we had to start with my diet, because my stomach was my biggest complaint. I was eating a lot of salads with my gluten-free diet (probably five days out of the week!), and he wanted me to reduce my salad intake and cut out coffee (I typically had one to two cups a day). Giving up coffee was hard! I was cranky and irritable for about two weeks; I couldn't sleep, and I had headaches. But Dr. Sinett was sure that the coffee was irritating my whole system and that anything I ate would give me pain until my system was soothed. So, I powered through, and very quickly, I noticed a difference. Even my face was back to normal—not puffy at all! I lost the eleven pounds I had gained instantly. My mood changed. Amazingly, I wasn't doing anything else differently; I had just reduced the inflammation in my body. Once my system was finally cleared, I could eat certain foods and tell right away what was hurting me. For example, having cut out salads, I drank a carrot-ginger-kale juice and swelled up immediately. If I have a big salad now, it gives me terrible cramps and sends me running to the bathroom.

Before meeting Dr. Sinett, I never would have thought that the gluten-free diet was bad for me. I thought I was eating healthy! I learned I benefit from a turkey sandwich much more than a kale salad. Kale is actually the worst food for my body. And that was my biggest lesson from Dr. Sinett: Everybody is different, and every person has different needs. The roughage and the acid from coffee are the things that are bad for me. I still eat vegetables, but I cook them. I incorporate small salads, take a multivitamin, and eat a lot of salmon, chicken, rice, and whole grains. When I eat, I listen to my body, and if I feel pain, it's a reminder of what I should avoid. Stress can really affect my stomach as well, and I often meet with a stress manager at Dr. Sinett's office. Sometimes, I'll have a glass of wine and feel great; sometimes, I'll have a glass and feel sick. Dr. Sinett taught me that drinking when you are happy can have a very different effect on your body than drinking when you are stressed. The food irritant coupled with the stress can seriously affect your health. These lessons—*don't follow the trends,* and *listen to your body*—have guided my life and brought me back to health.

All too many times, I meet patients who are like Sarah, and who are not tuned in to their body language—or who choose to ignore the bad things they are feeling because they are *sure* one of those diet plans is the "best" and should be working for them. Stress affects what you eat, it affects how you poop, and it affects everything in between!

6

Take Control of Your Shit!

Now you know the good, the bad, and the ugly as it relates to poop. Here are my tips for taking control of your body and bringing your input and output into a place of balance, so that you can have healthier and more regular bowel movements.

STEPS YOU CAN TAKE TO HAVE HEALTHY BOWEL MOVEMENTS

The basics required for healthy bowel movements (and a healthy digestive system) are fiber, fluids, exercise, and stress management. If your stool doesn't fit the profile of a healthy bowel movement, the following steps can make it better.

Eat Substantial Meals

Each time you eat a substantial meal, you stimulate stretch receptors in your stomach that are responsible for triggering normal and mass peristaltic waves throughout your small and large intestines. These natural contractile waves promote regular movement of waste material through your colon and rectum. Also, eating substantial meals allows significant boluses (roundish masses) of waste materials to travel together through your colon, turn into well-formed stools, and get eliminated from your body in an efficient manner. A substantial meal does not necessarily mean a large meal! Just enough to not feel hungry but still feel like you could run on a treadmill usually constitutes a substantial meal.

Don't Suppress the Desire to Go

Here's a tip for all those people who only like to poop at home and fight off the feeling when you are at work or elsewhere! If you regularly suppress the urge to have a bowel movement, waste materials spend more time than is optimal in your colon, causing excessive dehydration of these materials and formation of hard stools. One of the most common gastrointestinal complaints is hard feces and infrequent and difficult elimination—better known as constipation. If chronic, it may contribute to autoimmune diseases and colon or breast cancer. The longer stool stays in the colon, the more one reabsorbs some of the metabolic products (such as estrogen) that have been excreted in the bile.

Ensure Adequate Intake of Water or Water-Rich Foods

Water helps to move waste materials along and is absorbed throughout the entire length of your colon. Insufficient water intake can cause stools to form far before waste materials reach your rectal pouch, which can cause constipation.

This doesn't necessarily mean that you need to drink several glasses of water per day. If you eat plenty of water-rich plant foods, then you can rely on your sense of thirst to dictate how much water to drink.

Eat Fiber-Rich Foods Regularly

Fiber adds bulk to the boluses of waste material that travel through your large intestine, and this bulk is essential to your colon's ability to turn waste materials into well-formed stools.

A diet that is rich in vegetables, fruits, legumes, and whole grains ensures high fiber intake. Regularly eat foods that stimulate the flow of digestive enzymes, like brown rice, daikon radish, and pungent foods such as garlic, ginger, and onions.

Eat Fermented Foods

Eat fermented foods such as miso (fermented organic soybean paste), high-quality organic kefir, and pickles to replenish the beneficial bacteria in your gut.

Ensure Optimal Vitamin D Status

Optimal vitamin D status significantly lowers your risk of developing all types of cancer, including colorectal cancer.

Ensure Adequate Intake of Healthy Fats

All of your cells, including those of your large intestine and nervous system, require a constant influx of undamaged fatty acids and cholesterol to remain fully functional. If you don't ensure adequate intake of healthy fats, your nervous system and the smooth muscles that surround your digestive passageway—both of which are responsible for creating peristaltic waves throughout your digestive tract—may deteriorate in function. Also, intake of healthy fats is necessary for optimal absorption of fat-soluble vitamin A, which is critical to building and maintaining the mucosal lining of your colon. Foods that are rich in healthy fats include avocados, eggs, olives, extra-virgin olive oil, coconut oil, coconuts, raw nuts, raw seeds, and cold-water fish.

MINIMIZE GAS

There are a few ways that you can reduce gas. First, try removing common allergens from your diet such as wheat and dairy and see if you notice a difference.

If you do, you can add the food back in, but in limited quantities. You can also take digestive enzymes with each meal, either in food form or in supplemental form. Almost everyone finds that when they get their shit right, they minimize gas!

BUILD AND MAINTAIN A POPULATION OF FRIENDLY BACTERIA IN YOUR DIGESTIVE TRACT

Large populations of friendly bacteria can keep your digestive tract clean and healthy by:

- Promoting optimal digestion, thereby preventing build-up of toxic waste materials.
- Taking up space and resources, thereby helping to prevent infection by harmful bacteria, fungi, and parasites.

SQUAT

If you're daring, consider this: Squat on the rim of the toilet in your bare or stocking feet while you eliminate. "Squatting straightens the recto-anal angle and opens it more fully so elimination is much easier," says yoga practitioner Richard Ravizza, PhD, a psychology professor at Pennsylvania State University in Scranton. "You could think of it as straightening a partially kinked garden hose."* The Squatty Potty has helped many people achieve a better pooping position!

DE-STRESS

Movement and exercise can help with the digestive and elimination processes, as well as reducing stress, which many people hold in their stomach. Here are some exercise suggestions and other ways to reduce stress and potentially ease negative emotions and release them from being held in your gut!

- Get outside for a walk. Exercise does not have to be intense to be effective! In fact, if

* http://preventdisease.com/news/13/050913_A-Key-Predictor-of-Well-Being-Healthy-Bowel-Movements.shtml.

you have been training hard, take a day off from boot camp and rest!

- Get some sun and fresh air.
- Listen to relaxing music.
- Meditate or try other mindfulness practices.
- Get a massage.
- Take a hot bath.
- Take a few really good deep breaths.
- Laugh and let go.
- Snuggle a loved one or pet.
- Do yoga or stretching.
- Go for a gentle swim.
- Relax in a sauna.
- Have sex. (See? Who says nutrition coaching is boring?)
- Play. (Yes, play. Remember that? Play with your kids, grab a friend and a ball, or enjoy a game of *Pictionary*.)

Some of these things might not sound very effective, but what you have to remember about stress is that doing little things to free your mind for a few minutes can also help free your body of tightness and agitation. This, in turn, helps your muscles relax and gets your insides going again. It might not mean that you take one bath and get your shit back on track, but making time for one of these things every day, even for a few minutes, will help to regulate your body and balance your stress.

REDUCE ANTACIDS

People take antacids because they feel a burning sensation in their esophagus. The claim is that stomach acid backs up into the esophagus, but really, acid reflux is caused by inadequate production of stomach acid, which causes gases to rise up into the esophagus and create irritation. Doctors shouldn't prescribe you antacids without a test checking for stomach acid production. However, one in fourteen Americans takes antacids on a regular basis. So, how does this affect your shit? Not only do antacids not really fix the problem of esophageal burning in the long run, but they also create diarrhea because they contain magnesium. Some, on the flip side, have aluminum and leave people complaining of constipation. Usually, one way or another, people who take antacids complain of stomach cramps and changes in bowel movements.

Using these steps to identify things you are doing or *not* doing properly can help you have your "aha" moment about why you are having bad poops and can put you on the path to taking control of your shit!

7

What's in This Shit?

Healthy vs. Unhealthy: The Great Debate

We've learned that all foods are essentially both good and bad. Processed foods (foods in boxes, jars, and bags) are often only said to be bad for their added chemicals, fat, and sugar. However, there are a few benefits to occasionally eating some processed foods. By processing food, harmful bacteria is killed, and the way the food is packaged helps keep new bacteria out. It also allows for a longer shelf life. I believe it's important to stress the importance of the quality of the ingredients in an item because most of our choices are made right in the grocery store. The ingredients list for a kettle-cooked potato chip may just be potatoes, oil, and sea salt, but that will look very different than the ingredients on a Pringles canister! The same goes for microwave popcorn versus cooking kernels on your stove or using fresh ingredients to make your own pizza versus buying certain frozen brands.

The Good Shit

Okay, so what healthy foods are we eating that are misleading and may be a little more bad when we think they are a little more good? K. Aleisha Fetters, CSCS, author of *Fitness Hacks for over 50: 300 Easy Ways to Incorporate Exercise into Your Life,* gives a great no-bullshit list of no-good foods based on nutrition research—not corporate-funded studies!

Veggie Chips

Full of vegetables? Not really. They are made mostly of potato starch or corn flour. Usually, the only "veggie" you're getting is coloring from vegetable powders.

Granola Bars

Your granola bars may pack more than a third of your daily fiber needs in fewer than 200 calories by fortifying with extract of the chicory root. But most bars have added sugars, refined oils, artificial colors and flavors, and preservatives. There's a good chance that your bar is as nutritious as a candy bar—not a healthy meal replacement!

What's in This Shit?

Juices and Smoothies

"Even though they're packed with healthy nutrients like vitamins, minerals, and antioxidants, juices—even green ones—are loaded with sugar," says nutritionist Rania Batayneh, MPH, author of *The One One One Diet: The Simple 1:1:1 Formula for Fast and Sustained Weight Loss*. "Juicing extracts all of the fiber in fruits and vegetables that help you feel full and condenses a large amount of sugar in one small bottle that's too easy to drink in one sitting." Check the ingredients before downing a juice or smoothie to make sure it has fewer than 15 grams of carbohydrates per serving. Ideally, it should only contain one serving of fruit. The rest should be veggies.

Bottled Green Juices

While green juices sound like salad in a cup, you're likely getting more sugar than anything else. Some juices pack upwards of 50 grams of sugar per bottle, mostly from fruit. If you love your green juices, make sure you look for one low in sugar or make them at home in your blender!

The Good Shit

Frozen Veggie Burgers

Many frozen veggie patties are made from highly-processed soy or "textured vegetable protein," which is derived from soy and/or wheat—not veggies. It isn't so hard to make your own veggie burger with actual vegetables! Nutritionist Willow Jarosh recommends the Amy's Organic Veggie Burger and Veggie and Bean burgers.

Yogurt-Covered Snacks

Somehow, pretzels and raisins covered in shelf-stable icing has long been pawned off as "yogurt." Although the coating does contain an ingredient called "yogurt powder," it's mostly made up of sugar and palm kernel oil. That explains why some brands pack more than 15 grams of sugar into just six "yogurt"-covered pretzels!

Rice Cakes

Rice cakes may be low in fat and calories, but they're also low on nutrition (maybe 1 gram of fiber or protein with not much else!). Flavored versions just add artificial sweeteners, flavors, and colors.

Gluten-Free Snacks

"When you remove the gluten out of a food product, you're taking away the ingredient that provides that delicious, chewy texture in breads, muffins, cakes, pasta, and more. To make up for the loss of flavor and texture, food manufacturers often add in other fillers, including sugars, fats, and other chemical additives," Batayneh says. "Ultimately, your gluten-free snacks end up with more calories and sugars and don't even taste as good!" Most alternative flours used to make gluten-free foods have just as many carbs—or more—than wheat does and sometimes don't offer any more nutrients, like fiber, vitamins, and minerals.

Unless you have celiac disease, it's typically best to stick to products made with gluten!

The Good Shit

Frozen Yogurt

Fro-yo may seem healthy, but even plain fro-yo has about the same amount of sugar as the most decadent flavors: Half a cup has around 25 grams of sugar—and that's before you add in the brownie bites! I still like to go out for fro-yo, but I consider it a special treat!

Sushi

Grabbing sushi is definitely better than going through the fast-food drive-thru, but the tuna, sea bass, and swordfish in sushi are high in mercury, so it's good to be conscientious and limit your intake of those rolls! I suggest sticking with salmon or going with cooked entrees like cod when you go for Japanese food!

Pre-prepared Salads and Salad Dressing

"If it comes down to chicken nuggets or a prepackaged salad, the salad is most likely healthier, but that doesn't mean it's necessarily healthy," Batayneh says.

What's in This Shit?

Many prepared salads from restaurants, airport terminals, and supermarkets don't come with a nutrition label but actually have more than 1,000 calories. The cheese, croutons, and meats have a lot of salt, and most restaurant salad dressings have tons of added sugar! Some commercial kale salads, for example, have 600 calories and 40 grams of sugar. That's more than some cheeseburgers! Look for salads with nutrition labels and always choose extra virgin olive oil and balsamic vinegar instead of bottled dressing.

Dried Fruit

Dried fruit is yummy, but it's loaded with sugar! A serving of dried mango, for example, has almost 30 grams of sugar. Dried fruit should be your dessert if you choose to incorporate it! Otherwise, enjoy fresh fruit instead!

Anything "Sugar-Free"

Artificial sweeteners are bad for you. It's that simple. Aspartame is linked to cancer, and agave, which is supposed to be healthy, is very high in fructose. It's better to use no sugar or just a little bit of regular sugar if needed.

Yogurt

Plain or natural-flavored yogurt is a much better choice than the fruity flavors, which usually have sugary jam mixed in and not real fruit.

Low-Fat Foods

Low-fat/fat-free foods can contain up to 10 percent more calories and 40 percent more sugar. Fat adds flavor, so when fat is removed, companies need to add additional flavors and sugar to make up for the lost taste. This is especially true for those low-fat muffins at coffee shops that always look so good! They typically have less butter, but often have more sugar!

Instant Oatmeal

Oatmeal is a hearty, fill-your-belly breakfast. But some of those instant oatmeal packets contain 12 or more grams of sugar, while a homemade bowl of oatmeal of similar size may contain just 1 gram of sugar!

Microwave Popcorn

Microwave popcorn may contain potential carcinogens, as well as loads of butter and salt! Air-popped or stove-popped popcorn is much healthier, and lets you control how much you flavor it!

Iced Tea

If you make iced tea at home, it should have zero calories. However, when you buy store-bought tea, it's almost always sweetened with tons of sugar or aspartame!

Soy

Soy is high in protein and potassium and low in cholesterol. Not so bad, right? Well, when you choose a chocolate- or vanilla-flavored soymilk, it can be more like dessert with all the added sugar! Make sure to stick with unsweetened or plain varieties for your everyday drinking instead.

The Good Shit

Energy Drinks

Energy drinks promise to give you a boost with caffeine, vitamins, and minerals. But many of them aren't actually that healthy for you. I encourage my patients to drink water to rehydrate and enjoy a balanced diet. There's no better fuel!

Wraps

You may remember the early 2000s when anything in a wrap became a "health food." The problem is, restaurant-sized tortillas usually contain 400 to 800 calories. I like to go with a bowl instead.

Canned Soups

Canned soups are convenient and filling, but most have tons of salt. High levels of sodium can raise blood pressure and cause bloating, so I prefer to make a huge pot of soup from scratch. You can always freeze small portions to defrost for a quick meal!

What's in This Shit?

Wheat Bread

Wheat bread products can be misleading. Many wheat breads are actually mostly white bread with just a little wheat flour mixed in for marketing. Make sure your bread says "100 percent whole wheat" and that it has at least 2 grams of fiber—another mark of a truly healthy bread!

Pretzels

Pretzels may be better than greasy potato chips, but they still don't have much nutritional value. They are made with white flour, which quickly converts to sugar in your bloodstream, and don't really fill you up. I still like to have them but dip them in hummus to add protein and fiber.

Roasted Nuts

Nuts are a wonderful health food when eaten in moderation. But roasted nuts are just covered in sugar and salt. Try to limit your nut consumption to plain raw nuts. Or you can make your own roasted nuts in the oven with spices like turmeric, pepper, or even hot sauce! Yum!

Twig and Flake Cereals

Only healthy, right? Just because a cereal is organic, made with whole grains, high in fiber, or studded with flax seeds doesn't mean it's automatically good for you. Organic sugar is still sugar—and a lot of organic cereals pack just as much of the sweet stuff as conventional brands. Don't be fooled by high-fiber cereals, either: They're frequently supplemented with added fiber (read: not as absorbable) to make up for the fact that they're full of overprocessed, refined grains, says Kari Ikemoto Exter, RD, a registered dietitian with HealthCare Partners medical group in Southern California.

If you have been having diarrhea or constipation and have been eating lots of these foods, it's probable that these are some of your food irritants. In your bowel journal, make note of how often you consume these items, how you feel after, and what types of bowel movements they produce. Then try removing these things from your diet and note any changes. Low-fat foods don't really help your weight if they cause you to be blocked up!

So, what could you be eating more of, that our society has you avoiding? Here are some surprising healthier foods to try eating more of.

As we move away from the philosophy that all fats and carbs are bad, I'd like to point out a few foods that get a bad rap in dieter's handbooks, but actually are healthy in moderation.

Peanut Butter

Peanut butter may be high in fat, but 80 percent of that fat comes from healthy monounsaturated and polyunsaturated oils. Peanut butter is high in protein, vitamin E, niacin, folic acid, magnesium, and antioxidants. Natural peanut butter made from nothing but ground peanuts is the best, but if you buy commercial peanut butter, look at the ingredients and choose one that doesn't have trans fats, high fructose corn syrup, or much sodium.

Egg Yolks

Lots of people eat egg-white omelets to cut out fat, but egg yolks are an excellent source of choline, an anti-inflammatory nutrient essential for neurological function. Choline also helps produce the "happiness" hormones: serotonin, dopamine, and norepinephrine. Egg yolks are rich in lutein and zeaxanthin, two carotenoids that protect against vision loss. Despite this, egg yolks are high in cholesterol so you should moderate your intake and keep to no more than four yolks a week.

Bananas

Bananas often get poo-pooed because they're high in carbohydrates and calories relative to other fruits. But bananas have a low glycemic load, an estimate of a food's ability to raise blood glucose levels after a meal. They are low in fat and sodium, and have tons of potassium, vitamin A, folic acid, and fiber. I recommend eating half a banana, the equivalent of one serving.

Cold Cuts

Deli meat can sometimes have too much added salt and preservatives, but choosing brands low in sodium and saturated fat can make for a really healthy meal! I also recommend avoiding nitrates, which are added to preserve color and shelf life but can pose a cancer risk over time and suggest buying meat that is antibiotic and synthetic hormone free. I typically purchase Applegate ham, turkey, and bacon because it meets all of these requirements, and avoid meats like salami that are high in saturated fat.

Beer

Beer is equated with beer bellies, but beer in moderation can actually be good for you. It has no fat, cholesterol, or nitrates—and is loaded with significant amounts of carbohydrates, magnesium, selenium, potassium, phosphorus, iron, calcium, biotin, folic acid, niacin, B-vitamins, and antioxidants. (Ales typically have more antioxidants than lagers.) Moderate beer drinking can lower the risk of heart disease and stroke. What is moderate? One drink per day for women and up to two drinks for men.

Bread

100 percent whole grain is a home run. Whole grains have every part of the kernel—the bran, the germ, and the starchy endosperm. Refined breads are missing the bran and germ, where most of the vitamins, minerals, protein, and fiber occur. That's why whole grain bread always has lots of fiber—20 percent or more of the daily value!

Cow's Milk

Cow's milk has 8 grams of protein per cup while those alternative milks, like rice, almond, coconut, oat, and hemp milk, have only 1 gram of protein per cup. Cow's milk also provides about a third of the daily requirement for vitamin D and calcium, two nutrients that can be difficult to find elsewhere. Unless you are lactose intolerant, regular old milk is a healthy choice!

Potatoes

With low-carb diets being so popular for the last two decades, potatoes have been on the list of foods to avoid for quite some time. But potatoes are really one of the most nutritious foods on the planet. For 160 calories, they provide a feeling of fullness, as well as many nutrients including potassium, fiber, vitamin C, calcium, and magnesium. The potato can be a great source of carbohydrates and nutrients, including vitamins C and B-6, folate, and fiber (4 grams when you eat the skin). So, eat up that yummy potatoey goodness—just scrub it before cooking to remove dirt, pesticides, and other residues. Also, bake and roast potatoes, rather than boil, because the nutrients leach into the cooking water.

The key to keeping potatoes healthy is to eat the right portion size. Limit your portion to one small potato, or half or even a third of a large one. My favorite way to enjoy potatoes in a healthy way is to cut them into 1-inch thick slices, season with garlic, herbs, and pepper, and bake in the oven until soft and golden brown.

Canned Beans

Beans are packed with protein, fiber, B vitamins, and a load of minerals—and also are low in fat and sugar. And they're inexpensive. But who wants to soak beans overnight and cook them for forty-five minutes? No one! Canned beans, however, are a no-no because of the outrageous amount of added sodium. So, what to do? I buy low-sodium varieties and rinse the drained beans under running water for one minute, which rinses off that extra added salt!

Red Meat

Red meat is high in protein, iron, vitamin B-12, and zinc. Not all red meats make healthful choices (beef brisket, for example, has 16 grams of fat per three-ounce serving), but some varieties, like extra lean ground sirloin, can be up to 96 percent fat-free. My favorite lean cuts of beef are top round, top sirloin, bottom round, tenderloin, and flank steak. Research has also shown that grass-fed beef is lower in saturated fat and higher in omega-3s than traditional beef. Red meat once or twice a week, in appropriate portions (approximately a four-ounce serving), is healthy and satisfying!

Shrimp

Another healthy protein source is shrimp. While four ounces of shrimp does have 165 milligrams of cholesterol, it also packs 18 grams of protein and only a single gram of fat. When you enjoy a high-fiber breakfast and a meatless lunch, you should be able to fit shrimp into your diet and still come under your daily limit of 300 milligrams of cholesterol per day. I love it in homemade stir-fries, pasta, or just straight off the grill. Just avoid fried shrimp to keep this choice a healthful one!

The Good Shit

Iceberg Lettuce

Iceberg lettuce may not be as nutrient rich as darker greens, but it is far from being a pointless food. "It's nothing but water," people say. But aren't we all trying to take in just a bit more water? Water-rich foods help you feel full longer, and iceberg is extremely low in calories, so it makes a great base to load up with lean proteins like beans and seeds or fresh and dried fruits.

Rice and Corn

Rice and corn have been put down for having little nutritional value, and yet cultures have existed for thousands of years with white rice being their staple food! Those cultures are often considered quite healthy in terms of ailments and disease. Rice and corn are whole foods that can be very healthful in moderation, for most!

BONUS: SNEAK IN SOME SALT

While much of this chapter has pointed out products with added salt and have warned you about unconscious overconsumption, it *is* important to have some salt in our diets. Not everything should be low-salt and you shouldn't be afraid to add some to those yummy roasted potatoes. The problem lies in those products that have secret salt, which adds up to be too much!

My experience with most of my patients is that when they stop eating diet food and start eating real whole foods in healthy proportions with a proper carb, protein, produce ratio, they start having much healthier bowel movements. There are always exceptions, especially those with food allergies or more sensitive colons. A small steak with potatoes and an iceberg wedge salad with a sprinkle of blue cheese could be exactly what your body needs to get your system into a state of homeostasis. Now, doesn't this sound like a good diet plan? And one you can stick with?

A BIG (AND SOMETIMES DEADLY) CASE OF THE SHITS

Foodborne illness: Should we fear it?

Here's a question for you. Which is deadlier: lettuce or Doritos?

Well, lettuce has caused health outbreaks and even deaths recently, whereas Dorito intake hasn't had any immediate casualties, even though long-term consumption may be to your detriment!

Foodborne illness is one of the great terrors when it comes to creating epically bad shits. It seems like we are constantly hearing about E. coli outbreaks caused by consumption of otherwise healthy foods, like lettuce! The news reports symptoms such as watery or bloody diarrhea, fever, abdominal cramps, nausea, and vomiting within three to four days after consuming the bacteria. Some of those who become ill even die. So, what should you know about E. coli to protect your guts and all the bad shit that comes from it? Here are some fast facts.

HOW BAD CAN IT GET?

Of the 187 patients for whom information was available for the 2018 Romaine Lettuce Outbreak (sourced from the winter growing in and around Yuma, Arizona), 89 (or 48 percent) were hospitalized, including 26 who developed a type of kidney failure called hemolytic uremic syndrome. Symptoms of this syndrome include fever, abdominal pain, fatigue, small unexplained bruises or bleeding, and pallor. Most people recover within a few weeks, and while no one died from this particular E. coli outbreak, some can suffer permanent damage or die from severe E. coli infection.

HOW DO I AVOID E. COLI?

To avoid E. coli infections, experts advise thoroughly cooking meat, avoiding unpasteurized dairy products and juices, avoiding swallowing water while swimming, and washing hands and produce regularly and thoroughly before you eat.

With romaine lettuce being the most recent, here are the other recent causes of diarrhea and beyond:*

- **Ground beef and turkey.** 156 people across ten states were sickened by eating ground beef in April of 2019, and between February and August 2018, more than 36 million pounds of ground turkey was recalled after tests revealed a strain of salmonella. The outbreak killed one person and sickened 111.
- **Eggs.** In the summer of 2010, more than 1,600 people got salmonella found in eggs produced by Hillandale Farms in Iowa, which voluntarily recalled approximately a half-billion eggs in fourteen states.
- **Celery.** A processing plant in Texas was shut down in October 2010 after four deaths were tied to listeria-infected celery produced at the site. The Texas Department of State Health Services ordered SanGar Fresh Cut

---

* https://www.cnn.com/2019/04/24/health/e-coli-outbreak-ground-beef/index.html.

> Produce to recall all products shipped from its San Antonio plant.

I think it's important not to live your life in fear of foodborne illness and to eat foods like eggs and lettuce, unless there is a declared issue at the present time. If we cut out everything that has ever had a time of infection, we will be down to very little on our consumption list! The takeaway from this chapter is to remind you that most foods are sometimes good, sometimes bad, and it just depends on how you eat them, how often you eat them, and how your body digests them! Start ignoring all the hype that tells you peanut butter has too much fat and start listening to what your body and your poop are telling you about how peanut butter (and all other foods!) makes you feel!

8

Getting the Good Shit!

So, how do we get started on the right path of eating in a way that will sustain our bodies and keep them functioning in a state of homeostasis for a long time? This chapter is all about how to get your body on track!

A MORSEL ON INTUITIVE EATING

As we continue this journey to gut and bowel health via nutrition, it's important to pay attention to a new fad in dieting, which is, interestingly, the anti-diet known as *intuitive eating*. Intuitive eating basically means tuning into your body's hunger signals to help control weight. Gaining awareness of your own actual hunger helps you overcome mindless eating, eating from boredom, and eating from emotional stress, among other things. You are therefore only eating when your body is actually in need of nourishment, and you reduce all the excess munching that leads to weight gain. Overeating is one factor that leads to stomach inflammation, as the digestive system gets inundated with more than it can efficiently process. Here are a few tips to keep you from overeating.

Use a Smaller Plate

Portion sizes can play a big role in your digestion. Things such as super-sized fries or all-you-can-eat buffets cause us to overeat. Eating a pasta portion in Italy is very different than eating a never-ending pasta bowl at the Olive Garden. In Italy, pasta is frequently served on an appetizer-size plate. While on vacation in France, my family and I went to a supermarket and found a frozen pizza with pepperoni and sausage in an extra-large size called "The Big American."

In the past century, our plate size has increased by 22 percent and that has a direct impact on the amount of food that we are eating. Studies have shown that by switching to smaller plates we consume fewer calories. *Cooking Light* reported in August 2016 that by switching to plates that were nine inches in diameter as opposed to twelve inches, people consumed 250 fewer calories on a meal of grilled salmon, vegetables, and rice. If this happened at each meal, you'd be down over one and a half pounds per week. This portion size is much healthier because it allows your meals to be properly digested, without backup.

Pass the Treadmill Test

The nutritionists in my office have created a guideline called the treadmill test to help prevent patients from overeating. At any point all throughout a day, you should be able to jog on a treadmill. You shouldn't be so full that you can't do this. Ideally, we want your hunger levels to range from 3 to 6 on a scale of 1 to 10. We never want you to be too hungry or too full. Bad dietary choices and portion sizes tend to occur when you are outside the range of 3 to 6.

Eat High-Quality Ingredients

There can be a wide range of responses to foods based on the quality of ingredients. Cheese made on a dairy farm may trigger a very different response than a homogenized pasteurized processed cheese. Potato chips made from potatoes, oil, and sea salt are very different from a chip made from 42 percent potato content, the remainder being wheat starch and flours (potato, corn, and rice) combined with vegetable oils, an emulsifier, salt, and seasoning.

This brings me to something often on the mind of the American: Why do Italians eat pizza and not have an obesity problem, but Americans eat pizza and do? In Italy, pizza is almost always made with fresh tomatoes, mozzarella, and basil with fresh dough. Here, it can be. But it can also be a stuffed-crust pepperoni and extra cheese pizza loaded with extra salt and preservatives. When comparing cultures, sometimes there isn't a difference in the type of food being consumed, but there is a difference in the quality of ingredients. Good-quality fresh ingredients are much more likely to satisfy you sooner, causing you to eat less and allowing your digestive system to function optimally.

Getting the Good Shit!

Slow Down

Chewing your food more slowly reduces the amount of air you swallow with the food (which causes bloating) and is linked to reduced food intake and smaller portions. Smaller meals can be very useful with both digestion and excretion, as well as weight loss!

Have Breakfast and Small Snacks

Eat something within one hour of getting up each morning to jump-start your metabolism and keep you from getting too hungry by midmorning. Also, have a healthful snack between meals each day to keep your stomach from going on empty, and reduce what you eat in one sitting during meals.

Create a Meal Structure

A lot of people don't realize that the body generally likes to have structure around mealtimes, and portioned meals with planned snacks coincide with ideal rhythm of the metabolism. A meal structure can help get you into a natural poop structure, just how your toddler always takes a morning poop! I find starting with a guided nutrition plan gives you the visual for what a day should look like and offers a starting point for how much to eat at a time. Of course, there's always an adjustment based on size, physical activity, and more, and this is where your own intuitive eating should really kick in. The most important thing for you to do is to be aware not only of how much and when you are eating, but also to take better inventory of your body's other digestive signals in addition to hunger.

HOW TO IMPROVE THE GRADE OF YOUR POOPS

Keep a Food/Shit Journal

Sometimes you don't realize how much all that grazing adds up until you see it on paper. It's always amazing when my patients comment that they didn't realize they were feeling stomach discomfort until *after* they started feeling better. Most people are eating not only without paying enough attention to hunger but also without paying enough attention to their body's other signals, like pain, bloating, gas, discomfort, and the quality of their bowel movements. Intuitive eating is essential in many ways as you go through the nutrition plans that follow. I've found that overeating can contribute to digestive distress, and listening to your own hunger can be the first step in modifying your eating habits in a healthier direction. It's also necessary to become supremely conscious of your body's signals after eating and use those to help guide your choices the next time you're ready to eat.

Journaling about your input and your output is the best way to draw real conclusions, self-diagnose, and revise your diet—and ultimately improve your output. It's best to take a few weeks to eat as you normally do and really track patterns. While it's understandable that you want fast answers and quick relief to your digestive issues, you want to be extra careful not to reach the wrong conclusion because there are many factors in finding the right foods for you. Just because you had one bad shit or bloating after a salad doesn't mean that salad isn't right for you. Remember to think about other things: What was your emotional state? What was the portion size? What was the meal that you had before it? How much alcohol did you have during the meal? What type of dressing or seasoning? Try the same food again a few days later, then try it again in a different portion size, then try it again when you are in a different emotional state and compare notes. Anything that causes a similar reaction under different circumstances is probably not great for you.

Intuitive Pooping

As you progress with your journey to achieving the perfect poops, identifying good poops will become very easy, as will identifying which foods make you feel good. For me, a huge part of intuitive eating is being in tune with your pooping and other signs of your body that tell you if it likes what you are eating or not. Remember, if your body likes what you are eating, it is eliminating properly—and that keeps you feeling good and invested with the entire digestive process, from start to finish!

What to Write in Your Journal?

As you begin your journey to intuitive eating and more perfect pooping, track your input and output for about two weeks. Instead of ignoring signs of bloating, discomfort, or rushing out of the bathroom after a bout of diarrhea, take the time to sit with your journal and really document how you feel, what you ate, how much you ate, and how you were feeling emotionally at the time you consumed the food.

Blank pages are included at the back of this book to give you a place to keep notes of your daily input and output. Here is a guide to what to write as you record your journal upon completion of this book:

The Good Shit

INPUT RECORD

Breakfast

What I ate: ....

....

How much I ate: ....

....

How I felt after eating (pain/gas/bloating/discomfort?):

....

....

Lunch

What I ate: ....

....

How much I ate: ....

....

How I felt after eating (pain/gas/bloating/discomfort?):

....

....

Dinner

What I ate: ....

....

Getting the Good Shit!

How much I ate: ....

....

How I felt after eating (pain/gas/bloating/discomfort?):

....

....

Snacks/Drinks

What I consumed: ....

....

How much I consumed: ....

....

How I felt after consumption (pain/gas/bloating/discomfort?): ....

....

Today's Emotions: ....

....

....

OUTPUT RECORD

Bowel Movements

When did I go? ....

Ease and number of bowel movements: ....

....

What type on the Bristol Stool Chart?

....

Did I feel better after going? Was my stomach still upset? ....

....

Self-Assessment

After at least ten days of recording in your journal, go back through all of the entries with a highlighter, and look for patterns in input, output, and overall feelings of discomfort. The highlighter will help you easily identify repeats in input and output and indicate where you should begin changing your diet.

As you begin to understand how your body is responding to the foods you eat, it's time to start changing shit up!

The following are different directions for you to start with, depending on your current nutrition. I find most of my patients have success by following either a Digestive Rest plan, a Paleo Plus plan, or a

FODMAPS plan. Using your highlights from your journal, figure out which of these starting points you most identify with and follow with the suggested guidelines for that nutrition plan. Follow the plan for ten days to three weeks, continuing with the same entries in your journal.

IF YOU ARE A HEALTH FREAK, START WITH DIGESTIVE REST

If your stomach is inflamed and you qualify yourself as a health nut, eating lots of raw, vegetarian, or other forms of "clean" foods, the ticket to resetting your body may be to eliminate all of your inflammatory foods for a short time (even just two to three days will help your intestines breathe, so to speak). Remove raw veggies, dairy, sugar, and alcohol and eat small servings of carbs, lean proteins, and cooked veggies with an occasional fruit serving to get the inflammation in your tummy to come down, or give your digestive system time to rest. Protein, healthy fat, and carbohydrates will keep your energy levels strong. You may notice you start pooping better during this time. Slowly add back in your favorite foods, one food group at a time, and see how they each individually make you feel. This will help you easily detect which food causes a shitty situation!

IF YOU DON'T EAT VERY HEALTHFULLY, START WITH PALEO PLUS

The Paleo Plus plan is designed to eliminate toxins from your system in order to make a difference in the way your body functions. I recommend doing a full two weeks to cleanse the system and, if you notice a difference, stick with the plan as best you can moving forward. If you go on vacation or binge during a holiday, coming back to the baseline plan will help you after a short period of "falling off the wagon."

The Paleo Plus plan will clean up your diet without going overboard on raw vegetables. Here are the things you are allowed to eat:

- Oats, quinoa, rice for sustenance
- Nuts and seeds, including nut and seed oils

and butters, unsweetened coconut, vegetable oils, olive oil, and flaxseed oil
- Protein, including chicken, eggs, fish (especially mackerel, lake trout, herring, sardines, albacore tuna, and salmon), and lean cuts of turkey, pork, and beef
- All vegetables, including starchy veggies
- All fruits
- Decaffeinated coffee and tea (unsweetened)
- Seltzer and water
- Some dark chocolate or potato chips for a treat

This means *no* enriched white flour products, gluten, hydrogenated oils, dairy, fruit juice, sodas, alcohol, caffeine, or sweetened beverages.

IF YOU'VE BEEN STRUGGLING WITH STOMACH PAIN AND BAD SHITS FOR A LONG TIME, START WITH THE FODMAPS PLAN

Some people are sensitive to certain types of carbohydrates called FODMAPS, and if your body is unable to digest them, they can cause gas, bloating, diarrhea, or constipation. This plan removes all foods that contain FODMAPS, or Fermentable Oligosaccharides, Disaccharides, Monosaccharides, and Polyols, to restore digestive balance and reduce irritating or painful symptoms. The FODMAPS plan still delivers a balance of nutrients and allows gluten-free breads and corn tortillas so that you can still have comfort foods (yay for French toast and tacos!) without the uncomfortable side effects.

Foods you can eat: Fruits, vegetables, eggs, meats, and fish, canned tuna, unprocessed cheese, unsweetened almond milk, nuts, seeds, and nut/seed butters, quinoa, brown rice, brown rice bread, corn chips and tortillas, brown rice bread, soy sauce and vinegar, chocolate and sorbet for dessert! Feel free to use condiments like olive oil, balsamic vinegar, maple syrup, salt, pepper, hot sauce, vanilla extract, ketchup (with no high fructose corn syrup), brown sugar, and spices!

Foods not to eat: Anything with gluten (bread, pasta, baked goods, even things like breaded chicken cutlets count), breakfast cereals, canned foods, microwave or frozen meals, packaged cakes, cookies, snack foods, and things like packaged meat products such as hot dogs and bacon.

TIPS FOR ALL THREE PLANS!

Don't Eat the Same Shit Day After Day

If you found that your highlighter was really busy, you can also begin by eliminating all "the repeats"—the foods and drinks that you eat in a repeated pattern that ultimately can overwhelm your digestive system and impede a good bowel movement. Bombarding your system with the same chemical makeup doesn't allow the body to repair and rest and provide the necessary variety that our body needs. Regardless of whether the "repeats" are deemed "healthy," such as a green drink, salads, or smoothie, too much of anything brings frequent digestive stress to the body because it doesn't allow different digestive enzymes in different concentrations to do their job. Instead, the same foods make the body digest the same way over and over again. Eating the same foods, even while on one of my nutrition plans, is not beneficial for your system. You want to have at least three different types of breakfasts, three different types of lunches, and three different types of dinners and rotate them throughout the week. Try to mix up the content so that for breakfast, for example, maybe one day you eat avocado toast, one day you eat a vegetable omelet, and one day you eat cereal with milk and fresh berries. This will help keep your body from getting overwhelmed by any one food. If you need help with variety for each of these plans, my book *The Back Pain Relief Diet* includes pages of recipes for each diet!

Apply What You've Learned

You may be resistant to integrating nuts or some avocado because you are afraid to gain weight. You might not want to do the digestive rest and eat a grilled cheese for lunch instead of your salad because it has carbs and cheese. Remember, foods that reduce inflammation and encourage a healthy bowel movement are foods that reduce bloating, the feeling of gassiness, and pass through you properly. If your body is efficiently ridding itself of its shit, you may even lose weight by getting rid of those so-called low-fat foods and adding in some carbs and fat!

Let the Shit Show You the Way

Stop letting your belly do the talking. Your shit is actually the best indicator of what your belly really wants! Continue documenting as you consume new foods and perhaps try things that you weren't previously open to. Your most important area of focus will be on your poop. This will help you understand how your output is evolving as you shift your input. The goal is to start having mostly great shits (a 3 or 4 on the Bristol Stool Chart). Once you achieve this, you'll be able to stop journaling and continue eating with the newfound understanding of what your stomach likes and what it doesn't. Sometimes it's even okay to add in small doses of foods you were eating at the beginning without disturbing the homeostasis you've created. Just be honest with how you are feeling and how you are shitting!

Finally Getting 3s and 4s?

Once your poops are getting mostly 3s and 4s on the Bristol Stool Chart, your body is finally getting what it needs to eliminate properly. Once you are eliminating properly, write a new entry in your journal.

First, how does your body feel? Specifically, your stomach? Your back? Your skin? Many of my patients feel improved stomach comfort, a reduction in back pain, and clearer skin. Why better skin? Skin is the major excretory organ, and good bowel movements detoxify the body, leaving less for your skin to do!

Next, how are your energy levels? How is your sleep? Maybe even step on the scale and see how your new way of eating and pooping has affected your weight. (You may not even feel as concerned with the number, though, now that your body is feeling its best!)

I'll bet by changing your shit, you've brought your entire body into homeostasis and have noticed so many more improvements than just what's in the toilet bowl!

Conclusion

Be the Shit!

It's vital to get to the root cause of why you may not be having great bowel movements consistently and regularly. Whether it's your medications, your stress, the food you are eating, or a medical issue with your colon, it's imperative to your whole-body health to start shitting more easily and more healthfully. Here are my fast takeaways to remember as you move forward with this new understanding of colon health and the body language relating to your poop:

- Slow down! Enjoy your food!
- Reduce portion size by a third. See if it helps you feel less bloated or gassy and results in better bowel movements. Feel free to add in snacks to keep you from going too long between meals and to keep your digestive juices running!

The Good Shit

- Chart your stress levels and take the time to de-stress daily! Even five minutes of breathing, walking, or meditating can help!
- Get your shit moving by exercising. Not too much and not too little, exercise in the right forms and amounts can help your digestion, your stress, and your overall well-being. Chart your exercise and how you feel after.
- Journal about how you feel after each meal and snack using our handy Good Shit Record at the end of this book. This is your body language telling you what is happening inside. It's time to stop ignoring what your body is telling you!
- Note your shits, using the Bristol Stool Chart. Make connections between the foods you ate, the stress you felt, the exercise you did, and the shits you are having.
- Change your diet. Mix it up, take out your repeats, and see what brings about the most awesome shits!

Be the Shit!

This book is really intended to set you free from the gas, the bloating, the runs, the constipation, and all of the other stomach and bowel complaints that so many of you are having. I hope that you are now armed with an understanding of why poop is important and are feeling motivated to change your health and your life! Take control of your shit and find just how good it feels!

Happy Shitting,

Dr. Sinett

The Good Shit Record

As you learned, keeping a record of your shits will help you identify patterns in what you are eating and how that corresponds to how you are going! You should be aiming to have 85 percent of your shits be Good Shits, meaning your poop is graded a 3 or 4 on the Bristol Stool Chart the vast majority of the time. This means that you should be keeping a Shit Record until 8-9 poops out of 10 are GOOD SHITS. You should also be paying attention to what meals resulted in these good shits and sticking with foods that optimize your personal digestive process to keep up the Good Shit for years to come!

INPUT RECORD

Breakfast

What I ate: ....

....

How much I ate: ....

....

How I felt after eating (pain/gas/bloating/discomfort?):

....

....

Lunch

What I ate: ....

....

How much I ate: ....

....

How I felt after eating (pain/gas/bloating/discomfort?):

....

....

Dinner

What I ate: ....

....

How much I ate: ....

....

How I felt after eating (pain/gas/bloating/discomfort?):

....

....

Snacks/Drinks

What I consumed: ....

....

How much I consumed: ....

....

How I felt after consumption (pain/gas/bloating/discomfort?): ....

....

Today's Emotions: ....

....

....

....

....

1
DAY

OUTPUT RECORD

When did I go? ....

....

Ease and number of bowel movements: ....

....

What type on the Bristol Stool Chart? ....

....

Did I feel better after going? Was my stomach still upset? ....

....

Did You Score a Good Shit?

YES / NO

2
DAY

INPUT RECORD

Breakfast

What I ate: ....

....

How much I ate: ....

....

How I felt after eating (pain/gas/bloating/discomfort?):

....

....

Lunch

What I ate: ....

....

How much I ate: ....

....

How I felt after eating (pain/gas/bloating/discomfort?):

....

....

Dinner

What I ate: ....

....

How much I ate: ....

....

How I felt after eating (pain/gas/bloating/discomfort?):

....

....

Snacks/Drinks

What I consumed: ....

....

How much I consumed: ....

....

How I felt after consumption (pain/gas/bloating/ discomfort?): ....

....

Today's Emotions: ....

....

....

....

....

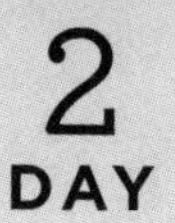

OUTPUT RECORD

When did I go? ....

....

Ease and number of bowel movements: ....

....

What type on the Bristol Stool Chart? ....

....

Did I feel better after going? Was my stomach still upset? ....

....

Did You Score a Good Shit?

YES / NO

INPUT RECORD

Breakfast

What I ate: ....

....

How much I ate: ....

....

How I felt after eating (pain/gas/bloating/discomfort?):

....

....

Lunch

What I ate: ....

....

How much I ate: ....

....

How I felt after eating (pain/gas/bloating/discomfort?):

....

....

Dinner

What I ate: ....

....

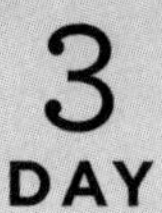

How much I ate: ....

....

How I felt after eating (pain/gas/bloating/discomfort?):

....

....

Snacks/Drinks

What I consumed: ....

....

How much I consumed: ....

....

How I felt after consumption (pain/gas/bloating/discomfort?): ....

....

Today's Emotions: ....

....

....

....

....

OUTPUT RECORD

When did I go? ....

....

Ease and number of bowel movements: ....

....

What type on the Bristol Stool Chart? ....

....

Did I feel better after going? Was my stomach still upset? ....

....

Did You Score a Good Shit?

YES / NO

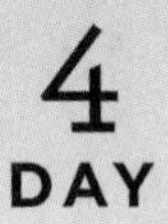

INPUT RECORD

Breakfast

What I ate: ....

....

How much I ate: ....

....

How I felt after eating (pain/gas/bloating/discomfort?):

....

....

Lunch

What I ate: ....

....

How much I ate: ....

....

How I felt after eating (pain/gas/bloating/discomfort?):

....

....

Dinner

What I ate: ....

....

How much I ate: ....

How I felt after eating (pain/gas/bloating/discomfort?):

Snacks/Drinks

What I consumed: ....

How much I consumed: ....

How I felt after consumption (pain/gas/bloating/discomfort?): ....

Today's Emotions: ....

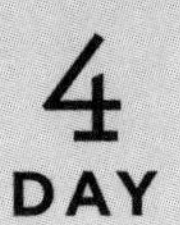

OUTPUT RECORD

When did I go? ....

....

Ease and number of bowel movements: ....

....

What type on the Bristol Stool Chart? ....

....

Did I feel better after going? Was my stomach still upset? ....

....

Did You Score a Good Shit?

YES / NO

INPUT RECORD

Breakfast

What I ate: ....

....

How much I ate: ....

....

How I felt after eating (pain/gas/bloating/discomfort?):

....

....

Lunch

What I ate: ....

....

How much I ate: ....

....

How I felt after eating (pain/gas/bloating/discomfort?):

....

....

Dinner

What I ate: ....

....

5
DAY

How much I ate: ....

....

How I felt after eating (pain/gas/bloating/discomfort?):

....

....

Snacks/Drinks

What I consumed: ....

....

How much I consumed: ....

....

How I felt after consumption (pain/gas/bloating/discomfort?): ....

....

Today's Emotions: ....

....

....

....

....

OUTPUT RECORD

When did I go? ....

....

Ease and number of bowel movements: ....

....

What type on the Bristol Stool Chart? ....

....

Did I feel better after going? Was my stomach still upset? ....

....

Did You Score a Good Shit?

YES / NO

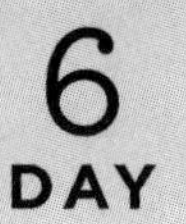

6
DAY

INPUT RECORD

Breakfast

What I ate: ....

....

How much I ate: ....

....

How I felt after eating (pain/gas/bloating/discomfort?):

....

....

Lunch

What I ate: ....

....

How much I ate: ....

....

How I felt after eating (pain/gas/bloating/discomfort?):

....

....

Dinner

What I ate: ....

....

How much I ate: ....

....

How I felt after eating (pain/gas/bloating/discomfort?):

....

....

Snacks/Drinks

What I consumed: ....

....

How much I consumed: ....

....

How I felt after consumption (pain/gas/bloating/discomfort?): ....

....

Today's Emotions: ....

....

....

....

....

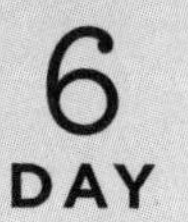

OUTPUT RECORD

When did I go? ....

....

Ease and number of bowel movements: ....

....

What type on the Bristol Stool Chart? ....

....

Did I feel better after going? Was my stomach still upset? ....

....

Did You Score a Good Shit?

YES / NO

INPUT RECORD

Breakfast

What I ate:

How much I ate:

How I felt after eating (pain/gas/bloating/discomfort?):

Lunch

What I ate:

How much I ate:

How I felt after eating (pain/gas/bloating/discomfort?):

Dinner

What I ate:

How much I ate: ....

....

How I felt after eating (pain/gas/bloating/discomfort?):

....

....

Snacks/Drinks

What I consumed: ....

....

How much I consumed: ....

....

How I felt after consumption (pain/gas/bloating/discomfort?): ....

....

Today's Emotions: ....

....

....

....

....

OUTPUT RECORD

When did I go? ....

....

Ease and number of bowel movements: ....

....

What type on the Bristol Stool Chart? ....

....

Did I feel better after going? Was my stomach still upset? ....

....

Did You Score a Good Shit?

YES / NO

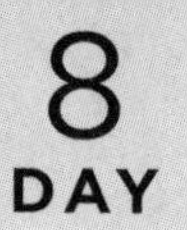

INPUT RECORD

Breakfast

What I ate: ....

....

How much I ate: ....

....

How I felt after eating (pain/gas/bloating/discomfort?):

....

....

Lunch

What I ate: ....

....

How much I ate: ....

....

How I felt after eating (pain/gas/bloating/discomfort?):

....

....

Dinner

What I ate: ....

....

How much I ate: ....

....

How I felt after eating (pain/gas/bloating/discomfort?):

....

....

Snacks/Drinks

What I consumed: ....

....

How much I consumed: ....

....

How I felt after consumption (pain/gas/bloating/discomfort?): ....

....

Today's Emotions: ....

....

....

....

....

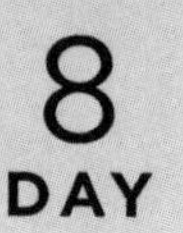

OUTPUT RECORD

When did I go? ....

....

Ease and number of bowel movements: ....

....

What type on the Bristol Stool Chart? ....

....

Did I feel better after going? Was my stomach still upset? ....

....

Did You Score a Good Shit?

YES / NO

INPUT RECORD

Breakfast

What I ate:...

....

How much I ate:..

....

How I felt after eating (pain/gas/bloating/discomfort?):

....

....

Lunch

What I ate:...

....

How much I ate:..

....

How I felt after eating (pain/gas/bloating/discomfort?):

....

....

Dinner

What I ate:...

....

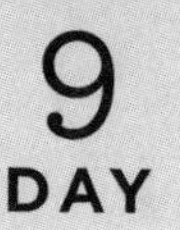

How much I ate: ....

....

How I felt after eating (pain/gas/bloating/discomfort?):

....

....

Snacks/Drinks

What I consumed: ....

....

How much I consumed: ....

....

How I felt after consumption (pain/gas/bloating/discomfort?): ....

....

Today's Emotions: ....

....

....

....

....

OUTPUT RECORD

When did I go? ....

....

Ease and number of bowel movements: ....

....

What type on the Bristol Stool Chart? ....

....

Did I feel better after going? Was my stomach still upset? ....

....

Did You Score a Good Shit?

YES / NO

10
DAY

INPUT RECORD

Breakfast

What I ate: ....

....

How much I ate: ....

....

How I felt after eating (pain/gas/bloating/discomfort?):

....

....

Lunch

What I ate: ....

....

How much I ate: ....

....

How I felt after eating (pain/gas/bloating/discomfort?):

....

....

Dinner

What I ate: ....

....

How much I ate: ....

....

How I felt after eating (pain/gas/bloating/discomfort?):

....

....

Snacks/Drinks

What I consumed: ....

....

How much I consumed: ....

....

How I felt after consumption (pain/gas/bloating/discomfort?): ....

....

Today's Emotions: ....

....

....

....

....

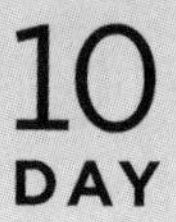

OUTPUT RECORD

When did I go? ....

....

Ease and number of bowel movements: ....

....

What type on the Bristol Stool Chart? ....

....

Did I feel better after going? Was my stomach still upset? ....

....

Did You Score a Good Shit?

YES / NO

How many good shits did you score out of 10?

Acknowledgments

The most heartfelt thank-you to Dr. John Procaccino for taking care of my mom, for taking care of me, for allowing me to interview you for my book, and for making this work your life's mission. The impact you have made on my life and on my family's lives will never be forgotten. It is my privilege to join in your mission to encourage as many people as possible to get colonoscopies before it's too late!

Index

Index

Index

Index

Index

Index

Index

Index